See Tarascon Publishing ordering information on page 192.
- *Tarascon Pocket Pharmacopoeia™ Classic edition*
- *Tarascon Pocket Pharmacopoeia™ Deluxe edition*
- *Tarascon Pocket Orthopaedica™*
- *Tarascon Internal Medicine & Critical Care Pocketbook*
- *Tarascon Adult Emergency Pocketbook*
- *Tarascon Pediatric Emergency Pocketbook*
- *How to be a Truly Excellent Junior Medical Student*

Tarascon Publishing®   Website: www.tarascon.com
Box 1159   E-mail: info@tarascon.com
Loma Linda, CA 92354   Phone: (800) 929-9926

"It's not how much you know, it's how fast you can find the answer."®

Important Caution Please Read This! The information in the *Tarascon Pocket Orthopaedica* is compiled from sources believed to be reliable, and exhaustive efforts have been put forth to make this book as accurate as possible. *However the accuracy and completeness of this work cannot be guaranteed.* Despite our best efforts this book may contain typographical errors and omissions. The *Tarascon Pocket Orthopaedica* is intended as a quick and convenient reminder of information you have already learned elsewhere. The contents are to be used as a guide only, and health care professionals should use sound clinical judgment and individualize patient care. This book is not meant to be a replacement for training, experience, continuing medical education, or studying the latest literature and drug information. This book is sold without warranties of any kind, express or implied, and the publisher and editors disclaim any liability, loss, or damage caused by the contents. *If you do not wish to be bound by the foregoing cautions and conditions, you may return your undamaged and unexpired book to our office for a full refund.*

Cover Artwork: *Muscles and Bones of the Human body,* Thomas Geminus, 1460. Courtesy of the National Library of Medicine, Images from the History of Medicine.

Tarascon Pocket Orthopaedica™
1st Edition

Damian M. Rispoli, M.D.
Staff Orthopaedic Surgeon
Malcolm Grow Medical Center, Andrews AFB, MD

Editorial Board*

David B. Carmack, M.D.
Assistant Professor of Orthopaedic
Surgery, R Adams Cowley Shock
Trauma Center, Baltimore, MD

Richard Howard, M.D.
Assistant Professor of Orthopaedics
St. Louis University

Steven M. Green, M.D., Professor of
Emergency Medicine & Pediatrics,
Loma Linda University, California

Mark D Miller, M.D., Associate
Professor of Orthopaedics, Chief of
Sports Medicine, University of Virginia,
Charlottesville, VA

Theodore W. Parsons III, M.D., Chairman
of Orthopedics, Residency Director,
Wilford Hall Medical Center, San Antonio,
Texas

Raymond Stefko, M.D., Chief of Pediatric
Orthopaedics, Wilford Hall Medical
Center, San Antonio, Texas

A Note from the Author
The *Tarascon Pocket Orthopaedica* is intended as a quick reference for Orthopaedic practice. It represents a compilation of facts and data that at one time I have had the occasion to need. It represents the basic information that was passed on to me from many talented individuals. If you find an error or wish to make a suggestion, please let us know (e-mail: editor@tarascon.com).

The author would like to acknowledge the helpful input and excellent review by the following individuals: Michael Gordon, MD; Bryan King, MD; Scott Nelson, MD; Felix Ungacta, MD; and Raymond Farrell, PA-C.

*Dedicated to Joshua, Zachary, Bethany, and Benjamin who sacrificed
many hours of Papa time to make this book a reality.
All my love and thanks to Vicki who really makes it all possible.*

Initial Approach to Trauma Assessment and Management

PRIMARY SURVEY

A Assess **Airway** (*immobilize cervical spine*)	• If poor or no air movement, perform chin lift or insert oral nasal airway. • Intubate if Glasgow coma scale ≤ 8, poor response to above, severe shock, flail chest, or need to hyperventilate. • Cricothyroidotomy or laryngeal mask airway if needed
B Assess **Breathing**	• Examine neck and thorax to detect deviated trachea, flail chest, sucking chest wound and breath sounds. • Needle chest for tension pneumothorax, apply occlusive dressing to 3 sides of sucking chest wound, reposition ET tube, or insert chest tubes (36 - 38 Fr) if needed. • Administer O_2, apply pulse oximeter, measure ET CO_2.
C Assess **Circulation**	• Apply pressure to external bleeding sites, establish 2 large peripheral IV lines, obtain blood for basic labs and type and crossmatch, administer 2L NS IV prn. • Check pulses, listen for heart sounds, observe neck veins, assess cardiac rhythm & treat cardiac tamponade. • Apply cardiac monitor, obtain BP, HR (pulse quality)
D Assess **Disability**	(Neurologic Status) • Measure Glasgow Coma Scale or assess if **A**lert, or respond to **V**erbal, **P**ainful, **U**nresponsive to pain • Pupil assessment - size, and reactivity
E Exposure	• Completely undress patient (but keep warm).

RESUSCITATION (Perform simultaneously during primary survey)

Reassess ABCD's	• Reassess ABCs if patient deteriorates. Address abnormality as identified, place chest tube if needed. • Emergent thoracotomy if > 1,200 - 1,500 ml of blood from initial chest tube, or > 100 - 200 ml/h after 1st h. • Administer 2nd 2L NS bolus, then blood prn. • Place NG tube & Foley catheter (unless contraindicated).

SECONDARY SURVEY

History	• Obtain *AMPLE* history
Physical exam	• Perform head to toe examination (including rectal/back).
X-rays	• Obtain cervical spine, chest, pelvic films, CT scans etc.
Address injuries	• Reduce/splint fractures, call consultants as soon as needed, administer analgesics, tetanus, & antibiotics prn.
Disposition	• Initiate transfer, admit, or ready OR. Document all findings, x-rays, labs, consultants, and talk to family.

Trauma Radiographs	Trauma history
Chest AP Pelvis Lateral Cervical Spine	**A** Allergies **M** Medications currently using (legal, illicit, and herbal) **P** Past illness/Pregnancy **L** Last meal **E** Events/environment related to the injury

Tension Pneumothorax

Chest pain, air hunger, respiratory distress, tachycardia, hypotension, hyper-resonant percussion, tracheal deviation, unilateral absent breath sounds, jugular venous distention (JVD), and cyanosis.

Emergent treatment: large bore needle into the 2nd intercostal space in the mid-clavicular line. Definitive treatment requires a chest tube.

Chest tube

Transverse incision 6th rib mid axillary line. Tunnel to 5th rib mid axillary line, place curved clamp into chest over the top of the fifth rib. Spread with clamp, insert finger into chest to clear area. Insert chest tube, secure in place, attach to pleurovac or Heimlich valve

Blood volume	Estimation of Systolic BP
70 kg man ~ 5 litres Child 80 - 90 mL/kg	BP ~ 60 mm Hg Carotid pulse BP ~ 70 mm Hg Femoral pulse BP ~ 80 mm Hg Radial pulse
Initial fluid management 1 - 2L in adult 20 mL/kg kids	<u>**Warm all IV fluids!!**</u>

Normal Acid Base Values

	pH	pCO_2	HCO_3
Arterial	7.37 - 7.43	37 - 43	22 -26
Venous	7.32 - 7.38	42 - 50	23 - 27

IV Maintenance Therapy (divided by 24 hours)

0 - 10 kg = 4 cc/kg/hr
10 - 20 = 40 cc/hr + 2 cc/kg/hr
> 20 kg = 60 cc/hr + 1 cc/kg/hr

Foley catheter

Assess prostate, scrotum, and perineum for signs of trauma. Consider retrograde urethrogram (RUG) in the presence of pelvic fracture or exam abnormality (blood at meatus, high riding prostate, severe pelvic trauma).

Shock = inadequate tissue perfusion

Cardiac Tamponade

> Beck's triad – venous pressure elevation, decreased arterial pressure,
> muffled heart tones. Echocardiogram or ultrasound may aid in diagnosis.
> Monitor ECG during pericardiocentesis, 16 - 18 gauge 6 inch needle,
> enter left and 1 cm inferior to xyphoid process, 45 degrees to the skin,
> advance while aiming at left scapular tip, aspirate as you advance.

American College of Surgeons Estimated Fluid and Blood Losses

	Class I	Class II	Class III	Class IV
Blood loss (mL)	≤ 750	750 - 1500	1500 - 2000	> 2000
Blood loss (%)	≤ 15	15 - 30	30-40	> 40
Pulse rate	< 100	> 100	>120	> 130
Blood pressure	Normal	Normal	Decreased	Decreased
Pulse pressure	Normal or increased	Decreased	Decreased	Decreased
Respiratory rate	14 - 20	20 - 30	30 - 40	> 35
Urine output (mL/hr)	> 30	20 - 30	5 - 15	Negligible
Mental status	Slightly anxious	Mildly Anxious	Anxious Confused	Confused Lethargic
Fluid replacement (3:1 rule)	Crystalloid	Crystalloid	Crystalloid Blood	Crystalloid Blood

Krantz, BE. (ed.) Advanced Trauma Life Support for Doctors, Student Course Manual. 6th ed. Chicago IL,
American College of Surgeons, 1997, p. 98.

Systemic Responses to Blood Loss

System	< 25% Loss	25 - 40% Loss	> 45% Loss
Cardiac	Weak & thready pulse, increased heart rate	Increased heart rate	Hypotension, tachy or bradycardia
CNS	Lethargic, irritable, confused	Decreased LOC and pain response	Comatose
Skin	Cool, clammy	Cyanosis, decreased cap refill, Cold skin	Pale, cold
Kidneys	Increased specific gravity Decreased urine output	Minimal urine output	No urine output

American College of Surgeons Pediatric Vital Signs

Age	Wt. (kg)	Heart Rate bpm	Blood Pressure mmHg	Respiratory rate /min	Urine Output mL/kg/hr
0 - 6 mo.	3 - 6	160 -180	60 - 80	60	2
Infant	12	160	80	40	1.5
Presch	16	120	90	30	1
Adol.	35	100	100	20	0.5

Krantz, BE. (ed.) Advanced Trauma Life Support for Doctors, Student Course Manual. 6th ed. Chicago IL,
American College of Surgeons, 1997, p. 297.

Pediatric Verbal Score

V-score	Verbal Response
5	Appropriate words or social smile, fixes and follows
4	Cries, consolable
3	Persistently irritable
2	Restless, agitated
1	None

Krantz, BE. (ed.) Advanced Trauma Life Support for Doctors, Student Course Manual. 6th ed. Chicago IL, American College of Surgeons, 1997, p. 304.

Glasgow Coma Scale

Eye Opening	Best Verbal	Best Motor
4. Spontaneous	5. Oriented, converses	6. Obeys commands
3. To verbal command	4. Disoriented, converses	5. Localizes pain
2. To pain	3. Inappropriate words	4. Flexion, withdrawal
1. None	2. Incomprehensible	3. Flexion (abnormal) decorticate
	1. None	2. Extension, decerebrate
		1. None

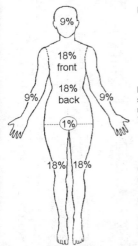

Estimation of Total Body Surface Area Burned

Fluid Resuscitation in Burn Victims

Parkland Formula

Lactated ringers 4 ml/kg/%burn body surface area in 1st 24 hours + maintenance fluid, with ½ over 1st 8 h, & ½ over next 16 h

Carvajal's formula

Carvajal's solution 5,000 ml/m2 of burn + maintenance 2000 ml/m2 in 1st 24h, with ½ over the 1st 8 hours and ½ over the subsequent 16 hours.

Shoulder Girdle

Muscle	Nerve	Origin	Insertion	Spinal Segment
Trapezius	Spinal accessory	Spinous process C7 - T12	Clavicle, scapular spine, acromion	CNXI, C2,3,4
Latissimus dorsi	Thoracodorsal	Spinous process T6 - S5, ilium	Humerus, intertubicular groove	C6,7,8 (posterior cord)
Rhomboid major	Dorsal scapular	Spinous process T2 - 5	Scapula, medial border	C5 (root)
Rhomboid minor	Dorsal scapular	Spinous process C7 - T1	Scapula, medial spine	C5 (root)
Levator scapulae	Dorsal scapular	Transverse process C1 - 4	Scapula, superior medial	C5 (root)
Pectoralis major	Lateral & Medial Pectoral	Sternum, ribs, clavicle	Humerus, lateral intertubercular groove	C5,6,7,8 T1 (lateral/medial cord)
Pectoralis minor	Medial pectoral	Ribs 3 - 5	Scapula, coracoid	C7,8 T1 (medial cord)
Subclavius	Nerve to subclavius	Rib 1	Clavicle, inferior	C5,6 (superior trunk)
Serratus anterior	Long thoracic	Ribs 1 - 9	Scapula, ventral medial	C5,6,7 (roots)
Deltoid	Axillary	Lateral 1/3 clavicle, Acromion, lateral 1/3 scapula	Humerus, deltoid tubercle	C5,6 (posterior cord)
Teres major	Lower subscapular	Scapula, inferolateral	Humerus, medial intertubercular groove	C5,6,7 (posterior cord)
Teres minor	Axillary	Scapula, dorsolateral	Humerus, greater tubercle	C5,6 (posterior cord)
Subscapularis	Upper & Lower Subscapular	Ventral scapula	Humerus, lesser tubercle	C5,6,7 (posterior cord)
Supraspinatus	Suprascapular	Supraspinatus fossa	Humerus, greater tubercle	C(4),5,6 (superior trunk)
Infraspinatus	Suprascapular	Infraspinatus fossa	Humerus, greater tubercle	C(4),5,6 (superior trunk)

Arm region

Muscle	Nerve	Origin	Insertion	Spinal Segment
Coracobrachialis	Musculocutaneous	Coracoid	Humerus, mid/medial	C6,7 (lateral cord)
Biceps	Musculocutaneous	Coracoid - short head Supraglenoid tubercle - long head	Radius, radial tuberosity	C5,6 (lateral cord)
Triceps	Radial	Long head - Infraglenoid tubercle Lateral head & Medial head - Posterior humerus	Ulna, olecranon	C6,7,8 (T1) (posterior cord)
Brachialis	Musculocutaneous – medial Radial – lateral	Anterior humerus	Ulna, coronoid process	C5,6 (lateral posterior cord)

Forearm Region - Superficial Flexors

Muscle	Nerve	Origin	Insertion	Spinal Segment
Pronator teres	Median	Humerus, medial epicondyle, coronoid	Radius, mid lateral	C6,7 (medial & lateral cords)
Flexor carpi radialis	Median	Humerus, medial epicondyle	2 - 3rd Metacarpal bases	C6,7,(8) (medial & lateral cords)
Palmaris longus	Median	Humerus, medial epicondyle	Palmar aponeurosis	C7,8 T1 (medial & lateral cords)
Flexor digitorum superficialis	Median	Humerus, medial epicondyle, anterior radius	Middle phalangeal bases	C7,8 T1 (medial & lateral cords)

Forearm Region - Deep Flexors

Muscle	Nerve	Origin	Insertion	Spinal Segment
Flexor digitorum profundus	Median (anterior interosseous) - index/long, Ulnar - ring/small	Ulna, anterior & medial	Distal phalangeal bases	C7,8 T1 (medial & lateral cords)
Flexor pollicis longus	Median (anterior interosseous)	Radius, anterior & lateral	Thumb distal phalangeal base	C8 T1 (medial & lateral cords)
Pronator quadratus	Median (anterior interosseous)	Distal ulna	Volar distal radius	C7,8 T1 (medial & lateral cords)

Forearm Region - Superficial Extensors

Muscle	Nerve	Origin	Insertion	Spinal Segment
Brachioradialis	Radial	Humerus, lateral supracondylar ridge	Radius, distal lateral	C5,6 (posterior cord)
Extensor carpi radialis brevis	Radial	Humerus, lateral supracondylar ridge	3rd metacarpal base	C(5),6,7,(8) (posterior cord)
Extensor carpi radialis longus	Radial	Humerus, lateral epicondyle	2nd metacarpal base	C(5),6,7,(8) (posterior cord)
Anconeus	Radial	Humerus, lateral epicondyle	Ulna, proximal dorsal	C7,8 (posterior cord)
Extensor digitorum communis	Radial (posterior interosseous)	Humerus, lateral epicondyle	Extensor aponeurosis	C6,7,8 (posterior cord)
Extensor digiti minimi	Radial (posterior interosseous)	Common extensor tendon	Small finger extensor apparatus	C6,7,8 (posterior cord)
Extensor carpi ulnaris	Radial (posterior interosseous)	Humerus, lateral epicondyle	5th metacarpal base	C6,7,8 (posterior cord)

Forearm Region - Deep Extensors

Muscle	Nerve	Origin	Insertion	Spinal Segment
Supinator	Radial (posterior interosseous)	Humerus, lateral epicondyle, ulna	Radius, dorsolateral	C5,6,7 (posterior cord)
Abductor pollicis longus	Radial (posterior interosseous)	Radius, dorsal ulna	1st Metacarpal base	C6,7,8 (posterior cord)
Extensor pollicis brevis	Radial (posterior interosseous)	Radius, dorsal	Thumb proximal phalangeal base	C6,7,8 (posterior cord)
Extensor pollicis longus	Radial (posterior interosseous)	Ulna, dorsolateral	Thumb dorsal phalangeal base	C6,7,8 (posterior cord)
Extensor indicis proprius	Radial (posterior interosseous)	Ulna, dorsolateral	Index finger extensor aponeurosis (ulnar)	C6,7,8 (posterior cord)

Hand/Wrist - Thenar muscles

Muscle	Nerve	Origin	Insertion	Spinal Segment
Abductor pollicis brevis	Median	Scaphoid, trapezoid	Proximal phalangeal base, radial	C8 T1 (medial & lateral cord)
Opponens pollicis	Median	Trapezium	Thumb metacarpal	C8 T1 (medial & lateral cord)
Adductor pollicis	Ulnar	Capitate, 2 - 3rd metacarpal	Proximal phalangeal base, ulnar	C8 T1 (medial cord)
Flexor pollicis brevis -Superficial head	Median	Flexor retinaculum, trapezium	Proximal phalangeal base, ulnar	C8 T1 (medial & lateral cord)
-Deep head	Ulnar			C8 T1 (medial cord)

Hand/Wrist - Hypothenar muscles

Muscle	Nerve	Origin	Insertion	Spinal Segment
Palmaris brevis	Ulnar	Transverse carpal ligament, palmar aponeurosis	Ulnar palm	C8 T1 (medial cord)

Hand/Wrist - Hypothenar muscles

Muscle	Nerve	Origin	Insertion	Spinal Segment
Abductor digiti minimi	Ulnar	Pisiform	Proximal phalangeal base, ulnar	C8 T1 (medial cord)
Flexor digiti minimi brevis	Ulnar	Hamate, transverse carpal ligament	Proximal phalangeal base, ulnar	C8 T1 (medial cord)
Opponens digiti minimi	Ulnar	Hamate, transverse carpal ligament	Small finger metacarpal	C8 T1 (medial cord)

Hand/Wrist - Intrinsic muscles

Muscle	Nerve	Origin	Insertion	Spinal Segment
Lumbrical	Median (index & middle) Ulnar (ring & small)	Flexor digitorum profundus (radially)	Radial aspect of lateral bands	C7,8 T1 (medial & lateral cords) C8 T1 (medial cord)
Dorsal interossei	Ulnar	Metacarpal shaft	Proximal phalangeal base, extensor apparatus	C8 T1 (medial cord)
Volar Interossei	Ulnar	Metacarpal shaft	Proximal phalangeal base, extensor apparatus	C8 T1 (medial cord)

Hip Flexors

Muscle	Nerve	Origin	Insertion	Spinal Segment
Iliacus	Femoral	Iliac fossa	Lesser trochanter	L2,3,4 (posterior)
Psoas	Femoral	Transverse Process L1 - 5	Lesser trochanter	L(1),2,3,4 (posterior)
Rectus femoris (Direct * and indirect ** heads)	Femoral	* Ilium, anterior inferior iliac spine. **Acetabulum, superior rim	Tibial tubercle (patella)	L2,3,4 (posterior)
Sartorius	Femoral	Anterior superior iliac spine	Tibia, pes anserinus	L2,3,4 (posterior)

Hip Adductors

Muscle	Nerve	Origin	Insertion	Spinal Segment
Adductor magnus	Obturator (posterior) Sciatic (tibial)	Inferior pubic rami, Ischial tuberosity	Femur, linea aspera & adductor tubercle	L2,3,4 (anterior) L4,5 (anterior)
Adductor brevis	Obturator (posterior)	Inferior pubic rami	Femur, linea aspera/pectineal line	L2,3,4 (anterior)
Adductor longus	Obturator (anterior)	Pubic rami, anterior	Femur, linea aspera	L2,3,4 (anterior)
Gracilis	Obturator (anterior)	Inferior symphysis pubic arch	Tibia, pes anserinus	L2,3,4 (anterior)

Hip External Rotators

Muscle	Nerve	Origin	Insertion	Spinal Segment
Gluteus maximus	Inferior gluteal	Ilium, posterior to posterior gluteal line	Posterior femur (gluteal sling), iliotibial band	L5-S2 (posterior)
Piriformis	Nerve to Piriformis	Sacrum, anterior Sciatic notch	Femur, proximal greater trochanter (piriformis fossa)	S1,2 (posterior)
Obturator externus	Obturator	Ischio-pubic rami, Obturator membrane	Femur, trochlear fossa	L2,3,4 (anterior)
Obturator internus	Nerve to Obturator internus	Ischio-pubic rami, Obturator membrane	Femur, medial greater trochanter	L5 - S3 (anterior)
Superior gemellus	Nerve to Obturator internus	Outer ischial spine	Femur, medial greater trochanter	L5 - S3 (anterior)
Inferior gemellus	Nerve to Quadratus femoris	Ischial tuberosity	Femur, medial greater trochanter	L4 - S1 (anterior)
Quadratus femoris	Nerve to Quadratus femoris	Ischial tuberosity	Femur, quadrate line	L4 - S1 (anterior)

Hip Abductors

Muscle	Nerve	Origin	Insertion	Spinal Segment
Gluteus medius	Superior gluteal	Ilium, between posterior & anterior gluteal lines	Femur, greater trochanter	L4 - S1 (posterior)
Gluteus minimus	Superior gluteal	Ilium, between anterior & inferior gluteal lines	Femur, anterior border of greater trochanter	L4 - S1 (posterior)
Tensor fascia lata	Superior gluteal	Ilium, anterior iliac crest	Tibia, Gerdy's tubercle via iliotibial band	L4 - S1 (posterior)

Anterior Thigh

Muscle	Nerve	Origin	Insertion	Spinal Segment
Vastus lateralis	Femoral	Iliotibial line, greater trochanter, lateral linea aspera	Lateral patella (quadriceps mechanism)	L2,3,4 (posterior)
Vastus medialis	Femoral	Iliotibial line, medial linea aspera, supracondylar line	Medial patella (quadriceps mechanism)	L2,3,4 (posterior)
Vastus intermedius	Femoral	Femur, anterior proximal shaft	Patella (quadriceps mechanism)	L2,3,4 (posterior)

Posterior Thigh

Muscle	Nerve	Origin	Insertion	Spinal Segment
Biceps, long head	Sciatic (tibial)	Ischial tuberosity, medial	Fibular head, lateral tibia	L5 S1 (anterior)
Biceps, short head	Sciatic (peroneal)	Lateral linea aspera, lateral intramuscular septum	Tibia, lateral condyle	L5 S1,2(anterior)
Semi-membranosus	Sciatic (tibial)	Ischial tubercle, distal-medial	Tibia, anterior crest	L4,5,S1 (anterior)
Semitendinosus	Peroneal	Ischial tubercle, proximal/ lateral	Oblique popliteal ligament, posterior capsule, posterior medial tibia, popliteus, medial meniscus	L5 S1,2 (anterior)

Leg Muscles - Anterior Compartment

Muscle	Nerve	Origin	Insertion	Spinal Segment
Tibialis anterior	Deep peroneal	Lateral tibia	Medial cuneiform, 1st metatarsal	L4,5 S1 (posterior)
Extensor hallucis longus	Deep peroneal	Mid fibula	Great toe, distal phalanx	L4,5 S1 (posterior)
Extensor digitorum longus	Deep peroneal	Tibial condyle, fibula	Lesser toes, mid & distal phalanx	L4,5 S1 (posterior)
Peroneus tertius	Deep peroneal	Fibula, extensor digitorum longus tendon	5th metatarsal	L4,5 S1 (posterior)

Leg Muscles - Lateral Compartment

Muscle	Nerve	Origin	Insertion	Spinal Segment
Peroneus longus	Superficial peroneal	Proximal fibula	Medial cuneiform, 1st metatarsal	L4,5 S1 (posterior)
Peroneus brevis	Superficial peroneal	Distal fibula	5th metatarsal tuberosity	L4,5 S1 (posterior)

Leg Muscles - Superficial Posterior Compartment

Muscle	Nerve	Origin	Insertion	Spinal Segment
Gastrocnemius	Tibial	Distal femur, posterior medial and lateral femoral condyles	Calcaneus (Achilles tendon)	L5 S1,2 (anterior)
Soleus	Tibial	Fibula, tibia	Calcaneus (Achilles tendon)	L5 S1,2 (anterior)
Plantaris	Tibial	Femur, lateral femoral condyle	Calcaneus	L5 S1 (anterior)

Leg Muscles - Deep Posterior Compartment

Muscle	Nerve	Origin	Insertion	Spinal Segment
Popliteus	Tibial	Femur, lateral femoral condyle fibula, head	Proximal tibia	L5 S1 (anterior)
Flexor hallucis longus	Tibial	Fibula	Great toe, distal phalanx	L5 S1 (anterior)
Flexor digitorum longus	Tibial	Tibia	Lesser toes, distal phalanx	L5 S1 (anterior)
Tibialis posterior	Tibial	Tibia/fibula, interosseus membrane	Navicular, medial cuneiform	L5 S1 (anterior)

Ankle/Foot Muscles - Dorsal Layer

Muscle	Nerve	Origin	Insertion	Spinal Segment
Extensor digitorum brevis	Deep peroneal	Superolateral calcaneus	Lesser toes, proximal phalangeal base	L4,5 S1 (posterior)
First Plantar Layer				
Abductor hallucis	Medial plantar	Calcaneal tuberosity	Great toe - proximal phalangeal base	L4,5 S1 (anterior)
Flexor digitorum brevis	Medial plantar	Calcaneal tuberosity	Lesser toes, distal phalanx	L4,5 S1 (anterior)
Abductor digiti minimi	Lateral plantar	Calcaneal tuberosity	Base of 5th toe	S1,2 (anterior)
Second Plantar Layer				
Quadratus plantae	Lateral plantar	Medial & lateral calcaneus	Flexor digitorum longus tendon	S1,2 (anterior)
Lumbrical	Medial & lateral plantar	Flexor digitorum longus tendon	Extensor digitorum longus tendon	L4,5 S1,2 (anterior)
(Flexor digitorum longus & Flexor hallucis longus tendons)				
Third Plantar Layer				
Flexor hallucis brevis	Medial plantar	Cuboid lateral cuneiform	Great toe - proximal phalanx	L5 S1 (anterior)
Adductor hallucis	Lateral plantar	Oblique head - 2 - 4th metatarsal base, Transverse head - plantar metatarsophalangeal ligament toe 2 - 4	Fibular sesamoid	L5 S1,2 (anterior)
Flexor digitorum minimi brevis	Lateral plantar	Base of 5th metatarsal head	Small toe, proximal phalanx	S1,2 (anterior)
Fourth Plantar Layer				
Dorsal interossei	Lateral plantar	Metatarsal shafts	Base of proximal phalanx	S1,2 (anterior)
Plantar interossei	Lateral plantar	3 - 5 metatarsal shafts	Proximal phalanx medially	S1,2 (anterior)
(Peroneus longus & posterior tibial tendons)				

Shoulder

Approach/ Eponym	Interval - Muscle (nerve)
Deltopectoral - *Henry*	Deltoid (axillary) & Pectoralis major (medial/lateral pectoral)
Lateral	Deltoid splitting no internervous plane (5 cm limit)
Posterior	Infraspinatus (suprascapular) & Teres minor (axillary)

Proximal Humerus

Anterior	Deltoid (axillary) & Pectoralis major (medial/lateral pectoral) Medial brachialis (musculocutaneous) & lateral brachialis (radial)
Anterolateral	No true internervous interval Brachialis (radial) & Brachioradialis (radial)
Posterior	No true internervous interval; long and lateral head of Triceps superficial, medial head splitting deep (radial)
Lateral	No true internervous interval; Triceps (radial) & Brachioradialis (radial)

Elbow

Posterior	No internervous plane
Medial	Proximal - Brachialis (musculocutaneous) & Triceps (radial) Distal – Brachialis (musculocutaneous) & Pronator teres (median)
Anterolateral	Proximal - Brachialis (musculocutaneous) & Brachioradialis (radial) Distal - Pronator teres (median) & Brachioradialis (radial)
Anterior	Proximal - Brachialis (musculocutaneous) & Brachioradialis (radial) Distal - Pronator teres (median) & Brachioradialis (radial)
Posterolateral - *Kocher*	Anconeus (radial) & Extensor carpi ulnaris (posterior interosseous)

Forearm

Anterior - *Henry*	Proximal - Pronator teres (median) & Brachioradialis (radial) Distal - Brachioradialis (radial) & Flexor carpi radialis (median)
Dorsal – *Thompson*	Proximal - Extensor carpi radialis brevis (radial) & Extensor digitorum communis Distal - Extensor carpi radialis brevis (radial) & Extensor pollicus longus (posterior interosseous)
Ulnar	Extensor carpi ulnaris (posterior interosseous) & Flexor carpi ulnaris (ulnar)

Wrist

Dorsal	No internervous plane; Between 3rd & 4th dorsal compartments
Scaphoid – volar	No internervous plane; Flexor carpi radialis (median) & radial artery

Wrist (Continued)

Approach/ Eponym	Interval - Muscle (nerve)
Scaphoid – dorsolateral	No internervous plane; between Extensor pollicus longus & Extensor pollicis brevis (posterior interosseous)

Pelvis

Approach/ Eponym	Interval - Muscle (nerve)
Ilioinguinal	No true internervous plane
Extended iliofemoral	Superficial – Sartorius (femoral) & Tensor fascia lata (superior gluteal)
	Deep - Rectus femoris (femoral) & Gluteus medius (superior gluteal)

Hip

Approach/ Eponym	Interval - Muscle (nerve)
Anterior – *Smith-Peterson*	Superficial – Sartorius (femoral) & Tensor fascia lata (superior gluteal)
	Deep - Rectus femoris (femoral) & Gluteus medius (superior gluteal)
Anterolateral – *Watson-Jones*	No true internervous plane; Tensor fascia lata (superior gluteal) & Gluteus medius (superior gluteal)
Lateral – *Hardinge*	No true internervous plane; Superficial – splits Gluteus medius (superior gluteal) Deep – splits Vastus lateralis (femoral)
Posterior – *Southern/Moore*	No true internervous plane; Splits Gluteus maximus (inferior gluteal)
Medial - *Ludloff*	Superficial – No true internervous plane; Adductor longus & Gracilis (anterior division obturator)
	Deep - Adductor brevis (anterior division obturator) & Adductor magnus (sciatic (tibial) & posterior division of obturator)

Femur

Approach/ Eponym	Interval - Muscle (nerve)
Lateral	No internervous plane; Splits Vastus lateralis (femoral)
Anteromedial	No true internervous plane; Rectus femoris (femoral) & Vastus medialis (femoral)
Posterolateral	Vastus lateralis (femoral) & Hamstrings (sciatic)
Posterior distal femur	Biceps femoris (sciatic) & Vastus lateralis (femoral)

Knee

Approach/ Eponym	Interval - Muscle (nerve)
Medial parapatellar	No true internervous plane; Vastus medialis (femoral) & Rectus femoris (femoral)
Medial	No true internervous plane; Vastus medialis (femoral) & Sartorius (femoral)
Lateral	Iliotibial band (superior gluteal) & Biceps femoris (sciatic)
Posterior	Semimembranosus/Medial Gastrocnemius (tibial) & Biceps femoris/Lateral Gastrocnemius (tibial)

Leg

Approach/ Eponym	Interval - Muscle (nerve)
Anterior	No internervous plane; Tibialis anterior (peroneal) & periosteum
Anterolateral	Superficial - Peroneus brevis (superficial peroneal) & Extensor digitorum longus (deep peroneal) Deep - Tibialis posterior (tibial) & Extensor muscles (deep peroneal)
Posterolateral	Gastrocnemius, Soleus, Flexor hallucis longus (tibial) & Peroneus brevis and longus (superficial peroneal)
Fibula	Peroneal muscles (superficial peroneal) & Flexor muscles (tibial)

Ankle

Anterior or Dorsal	No internervous plane; Extensor hallucis longus (deep peroneal) & Extensor digitorum longus (deep peroneal)
To Medial Malleolus	No internervous plane; direct approach
To Lateral Malleolus	Peroneus tertius (deep peroneal) & Peroneus brevis (superficial peroneal)
Posteromedial	No internervous plane; Tibialis posterior or Flexor digitorum longus (tibial) & Flexor digitorum longus or Flexor hallucis longus (tibial)
Posterolateral	Peroneus brevis (superficial peroneal) & Flexor hallucis longus (tibial)

Contents of the Sciatic Notch
(Greater Sciatic notch)
<u>Above the Piriformis muscle</u>
Superior gluteal nerve
Superior gluteal artery
<u>Below the Piriformis</u>
Inferior gluteal nerve
Inferior gluteal artery
Pudendal nerve
Internal Pudendal artery
Nerve to the Obturator internus
Sciatic nerve
Posterior femoral cutaneous nerve
Nerve to Quadratus femoris

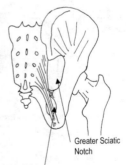

Greater Sciatic Notch

Lesser Sciatic Notch

PROXIMAL ARM CROSS SECTION
(anterior = top, right = medial)

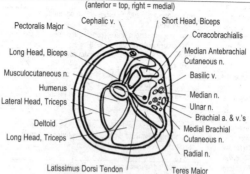

Pectoralis Major

Cephalic v.

Short Head, Biceps

Coracobrachialis

Long Head, Biceps

Median Antebrachial Cutaneous n.

Musculocutaneous n.

Basilic v.

Humerus

Median n.

Lateral Head, Triceps

Ulnar n.

Deltoid

Brachial a. & v.'s

Long Head, Triceps

Medial Brachial Cutaneous n.

Radial n.

Latissimus Dorsi Tendon

Teres Major

MID ARM CROSS SECTION
(anterior = top, right = medial)

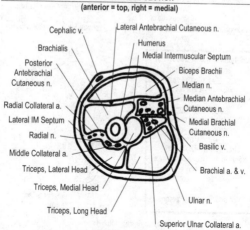

Cephalic v.

Lateral Antebrachial Cutaneous n.

Brachialis

Humerus

Posterior Antebrachial Cutaneous n.

Medial Intermuscular Septum

Biceps Brachii

Median n.

Radial Collateral a.

Median Antebrachial Cutaneous n.

Lateral IM Septum

Medial Brachial Cutaneous n.

Radial n.

Basilic v.

Middle Collateral a.

Brachial a. & v.

Triceps, Lateral Head

Triceps, Medial Head

Ulnar n.

Triceps, Long Head

Superior Ulnar Collateral a.

DISTAL ARM CROSS SECTION
(anterior = top, right = medial)

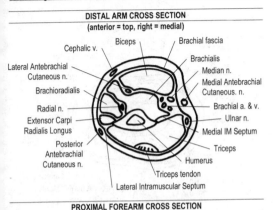

Biceps
Cephalic v.
Brachial fascia
Brachialis
Lateral Antebrachial Cutaneous n.
Median n.
Medial Antebrachial Cutaneous. n.
Brachioradialis
Radial n.
Brachial A. & v.
Extensor Carpi Radialis Longus
Ulnar n.
Posterior Antebrachial Cutaneous n.
Medial IM Septum
Triceps
Humerus
Triceps tendon
Lateral Intramuscular Septum

PROXIMAL FOREARM CROSS SECTION
(volar = top, right = ulnar)

Radius
Superficial Branch Radial n.
Radial a.
Medial Antebrachial v.
Pronator Teres
Brachioradialis
Medial Antebrachial Cutaneous n.
Cephalic v.
Lateral Antebrachial Cutaneous n.
Palmaris Longus
Flexor Carpi Radialis
Extensor Carpi Radialis Longus
Flexor Digitorum Superficialis
Extensor Carpi Radialis Brevis
Ulnar n.
Flexor Carpi Ulnaris
Radial n.
Flexor Digitorum Profundus
Extensor Digitorum Communis
Ulna
Anconeus
F P Longus
Median n., Ulnar a., & Common Interosseous a. (volar to dorsal)
Extensor Digiti Quinti Minimi
Supinator
Posterior Antebrachial Cutaneous n.
Extensor Carpi Ulnaris

MID FOREARM CROSS SECTION
(volar = top, right = ulnar)

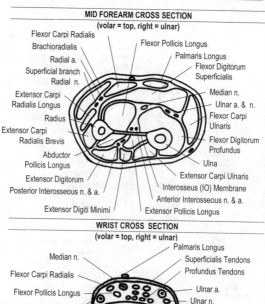

Flexor Carpi Radialis
Brachioradialis
Radial a.
Superficial branch
Radial n.
Extensor Carpi Radialis Longus
Radius
Extensor Carpi Radialis Brevis
Abductor Pollicis Longus
Extensor Digitorum
Posterior Interosseus n. & a.
Extensor Digiti Minimi

Flexor Pollicis Longus
Palmaris Longus
Flexor Digitorum Superficialis
Median n.
Ulnar a. & n.
Flexor Carpi Ulnaris
Flexor Digitorum Profundus
Ulna
Extensor Carpi Ulnaris
Interosseus (IO) Membrane
Anterior Interosseus n. & a.
Extensor Pollicis Longus

WRIST CROSS SECTION
(volar = top, right = ulnar)

Palmaris Longus
Superficialis Tendons
Profundus Tendons
Median n.
Flexor Carpi Radialis
Flexor Pollicis Longus
Ulnar a.
Ulnar n.
Flexor Carpi Ulnaris
Radial a.

Compartment 1
Extensor Pollicis Brevis
Abductor Pollicis Longus

Compartment 2
Extensor Carpi Radialis
Longus & Brevis

Compartment 3
Extensor Pollicis Longus

Compartment 6
Extensor Carpi Ulnaris

Compartment 5
Extensor Digiti Minimi

Compartment 4
Extensor Digitorum & Indicis Proprius

PROXIMAL THIGH CROSS SECTION
(anterior = top, right = medial)

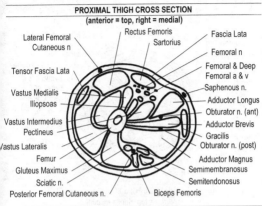

Lateral Femoral Cutaneous n.
Rectus Femoris
Sartorius
Fascia Lata
Femoral n
Tensor Fascia Lata
Femoral & Deep Femoral a & v
Vastus Medialis
Iliopsoas
Saphenous n.
Adductor Longus
Vastus Intermedius
Pectineus
Obturator n. (ant)
Adductor Brevis
Vastus Lateralis
Femur
Gracilis
Obturator n. (post)
Gluteus Maximus
Sciatic n.
Adductor Magnus
Semimembranosus
Semitendonosus
Posterior Femoral Cutaneous n.
Biceps Femoris

MID THIGH CROSS SECTION
(anterior = top, right = medial)

Femoral a. & v.
Saphenous n. & n. to Vastus Medialis
Vastus Medialis
Rectus Femoris
Sartorius
Vastus Intermedius
Adductor Longus
Vastus Lateralis
Adductor Brevis
Femur
Gracilis
Iliotibial tract
Great Saphenous v.
Biceps Femoris, short head
Adductor Magnus
Biceps Femoris, long head
Deep Femoral a. & v.
Semitendonosus
Sciatic nerve
Semimembranosus

DISTAL THIGH CROSS SECTION
(anterior = top, right = medial)

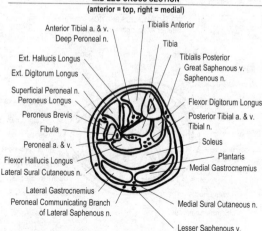

Q femoris tendon
Vastus Intermedius
Articularis genu
Iliotibial tract
Vastus lateralis
Popliteal a .
Popliteal v.
Biceps Femoris
Common Peroneal n.
Tibial n.
Semitendonosus

Vastus Medialis
Femur
Adductor Magnus tendon
Saphenous n.
Descending genicular a.
Sartorius
Great Saphenous v.
Gracilis
Semimembranosus

MID LEG CROSS SECTION
(anterior = top, right = medial)

Anterior Tibial a. & v.
Deep Peroneal n.
Ext. Hallucis Longus
Ext. Digitorum Longus
Superficial Peroneal n.
Peroneus Longus
Peroneus Brevis
Fibula
Peroneal a. & v.
Flexor Hallucis Longus
Lateral Sural Cutaneous n.
Lateral Gastrocnemius
Peroneal Communicating Branch
of Lateral Saphenous n.

Tibialis Anterior
Tibia
Tibialis Posterior
Great Saphenous v.
Saphenous n.
Flexor Digitorum Longus
Posterior Tibial a. & v.
Tibial n.
Soleus
Plantaris
Medial Gastrocnemius
Medial Sural Cutaneous n.
Lesser Saphenous v.

Arteries about the shoulder

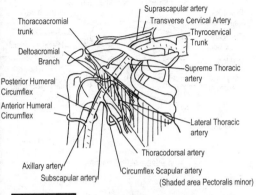

- Suprascapular artery
- Transverse Cervical Artery
- Thyrocervical Trunk
- Supreme Thoracic artery
- Lateral Thoracic artery
- Thoracodorsal artery
- Circumflex Scapular artery
- (Shaded area Pectoralis minor)
- Thoracoacromial trunk
- Deltoacromial Branch
- Posterior Humeral Circumflex
- Anterior Humeral Circumflex
- Axillary artery
- Subscapular artery

Arteries about the elbow

> **Radial to Ulnar at the elbow -- TAN**
> **Tendon-Artery-Nerve**

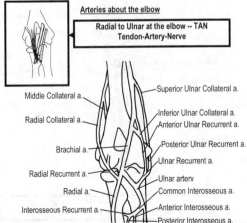

- Middle Collateral a.
- Radial Collateral a.
- Brachial a.
- Radial Recurrent a.
- Radial a.
- Interosseous Recurrent a.
- Superior Ulnar Collateral a.
- Inferior Ulnar Collateral a.
- Anterior Ulnar Recurrent a.
- Posterior Ulnar Recurrent a.
- Ulnar Recurrent a.
- Ulnar artery
- Common Interosseous a.
- Anterior Interosseous a.
- Posterior Interosseous a.

Shoulder Spaces and Intervals
(Posterior View of Shoulder)

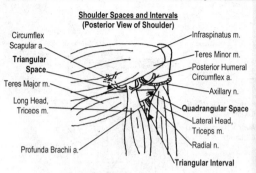

Circumflex Scapular a.

Triangular Space

Teres Major m.

Long Head, Triceps m.

Profunda Brachii a.

Infraspinatus m.

Teres Minor m.

Posterior Humeral Circumflex a.

Axillary n.

Quadrangular Space

Lateral Head, Triceps m.

Radial n.

Triangular Interval

Arteries of the Forearm

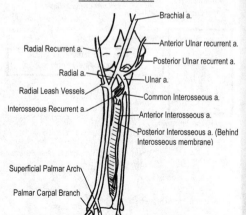

Brachial a.

Anterior Ulnar recurrent a.

Posterior Ulnar recurrent a.

Radial Recurrent a.

Radial a.

Ulnar a.

Radial Leash Vessels

Common Interosseous a.

Interosseous Recurrent a.

Anterior Interosseous a.

Posterior Interosseous a. (Behind Interosseous membrane)

Superficial Palmar Arch

Palmar Carpal Branch

Nerves frame the Wrist – (Radial to Ulnar)
Superficial Branch Radial n.-Radial a.-Median n.-Ulnar a.-Ulnar n.

Pelvic Arteries

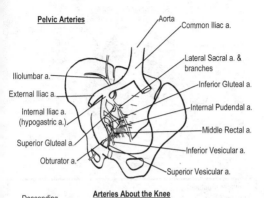

Arteries About the Knee

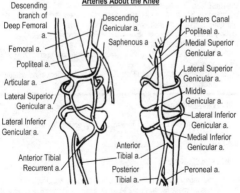

Anterior   Posterior

> Behind the knee – Lateral to Medial
> Nerve-Vein-Artery

Glenohumeral Ligaments
(Lateral disarticulated view)

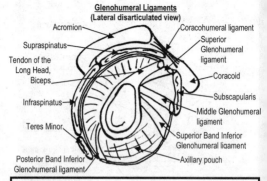

Acromion — Coracohumeral ligament
Superior Glenohumeral ligament
Supraspinatus
Tendon of the Long Head, Biceps — Coracoid
Infraspinatus — Subscapularis
Middle Glenohumeral ligament
Teres Minor
Superior Band Inferior Glenohumeral ligament
Posterior Band Inferior Glenohumeral ligament — Axillary pouch

---

Shoulder (Posteriorly)

<u>Triangular Space</u> – Circumflex scapular artery
<u>Quadrangular Space</u> – Posterior humeral circumflex artery, Axillary nerve
<u>Triangular interval</u> – Profunda brachii artery, Radial nerve

Axillary artery (divided into three parts by the Pectoralis minor muscle)
1. Supreme Thoracic artery (before muscle, 1 branch)
2. Thoracoacromial and Lateral Thoracic arteries (under muscle, 2 branches)
3. Subscapular, Anterior and Posterior Humeral Circumflex arteries (after muscle, 3 branches)

Medial Layers of the Knee[1]
I. Sartorius and fascia
II. Superficial medial collateral ligament, posterior oblique ligament, semimembranosus
III. Deep Medial collateral ligament, capsule

Lateral Layers of the Knee[2]
I. Iliotibial tract, biceps
II. Patellar retinaculum, patellofemoral ligament, popliteofibular ligament
III. Arcuate ligament, fabello-fibular ligament, capsule, lateral collateral ligament

---

[1] Warren LF, Marshall JL. The supporting structures and layers on the medial side of the knee. JBJS 61A:56-62, 1979.
[2] Seebacher JR, Inglis AE, and Marshall JL. The structure of the posterolateral aspect of the knee. JBJS 64A:536-541, 1982.

Volar Wrist Ligaments

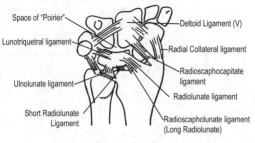

Space of "Poirier"

Lunotriquetral ligament

Ulnolunate ligament

Short Radiolunate Ligament

Deltoid Ligament (V)

Radial Collateral ligament

Radioscaphocapitate ligament

Radiolunate ligament

Radioscapholunate ligament (Long Radiolunate)

Elbow Ligaments

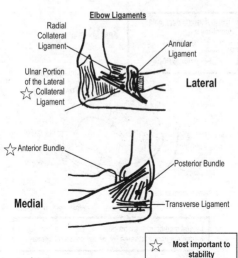

Radial Collateral Ligament

☆ Ulnar Portion of the Lateral Collateral Ligament

Annular Ligament

Lateral

☆ Anterior Bundle

Medial

Posterior Bundle

Transverse Ligament

| ☆ | Most important to stability |

Pelvic Ligaments

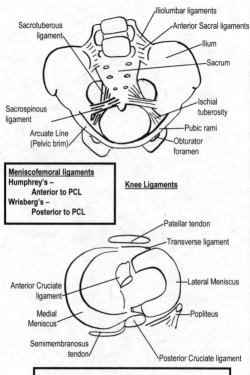

Iliolumbar ligaments
Anterior Sacral ligaments
Ilium
Sacrum
Ischial tuberosity
Pubic rami
Obturator foramen
Sacrotuberous ligament
Sacrospinous ligament
Arcuate Line (Pelvic brim)

Meniscofemoral ligaments
Humphrey's –
       Anterior to PCL
Wrisberg's –
       Posterior to PCL

Knee Ligaments

Patellar tendon
Transverse ligament
Lateral Meniscus
Popliteus
Posterior Cruciate ligament
Anterior Cruciate ligament
Medial Meniscus
Semimembranosus tendon

Lateral meniscus more mobile
Medial meniscus tethered by medial collateral ligament

Posterior Knee Ligaments/Tendons
(medial left, lateral right)

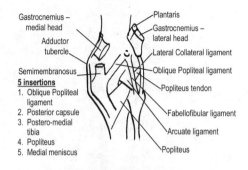

Gastrocnemius – medial head

Adductor tubercle

Semimembranosus
5 insertions
1. Oblique Popliteal ligament
2. Posterior capsule
3. Postero-medial tibia
4. Popliteus
5. Medial meniscus

Plantaris

Gastrocnemius – lateral head

Lateral Collateral ligament

Oblique Popliteal ligament

Popliteus tendon

Fabellofibular ligament

Arcuate ligament

Popliteus

Ankle Ligaments

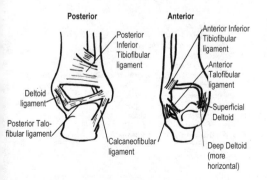

Posterior

Posterior Inferior Tibiofibular ligament

Deltoid ligament

Posterior Talo-fibular ligament

Calcaneofibular ligament

Anterior

Anterior Inferior Tibiofibular ligament

Anterior Talofibular ligament

Superficial Deltoid

Deep Deltoid (more horizontal)

FINGER EXTENSOR APPARATUS

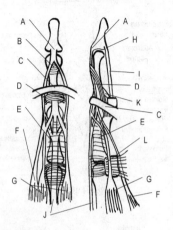

A. Terminal Tendon
B. Triangular Ligament
C. Transverse Retinacular Ligament
D. Conjoined Lateral Band
E. Oblique & Transverse Fibers of the Intrinsic Apparatus
F. Lumbrical Muscle (Originating on the radial side of the flexor digitorum profundus tendon)
G. Interossei Muscle
H. Flexor Digitorum Profundus Insertion
I. Flexor Digitorum Profundus Tendon
J. Extensor Digitorum Communis
K. Flexor Digitorum Superficialis Insertion
L. Sagittal Bands

FINGER PULLEY SYSTEM

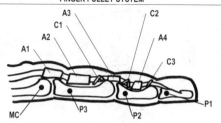

A2 & A4 most important, A1 released in surgical treatment of a trigger digit

NERVE PLEXUS

Brachial

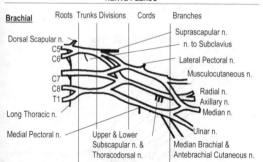

Trunks = Upper, Middle and Lower
Divisions = Anterior and Posterior
Cords = Lateral, Posterior, and Medial

Radial and Axillary nerves come off the
posterior cord, the sum of the posterior
divisions

Plexus Mnemonic –	Robert Taylor Drinks Cold Beer
	Roots, Trunks, Divisions, Cords, Branches
Posterior Branches	
Mnemonic -	STAR (Medial to Lateral)
	Subscapular (upper and lower surround Thoracodorsal n.)
	Thoracodorsal, Axillary, Radial

Lumbar

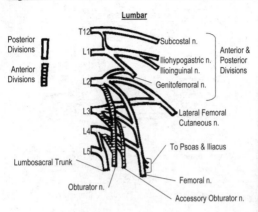

Posterior Divisions

Anterior Divisions

T12
L1
L2
L3
L4
L5

Subcostal n.
Iliohypogastric n.
Ilioinguinal n.
Genitofemoral n.

Anterior & Posterior Divisions

Lateral Femoral Cutaneous n.

To Psoas & Iliacus

Lumbosacral Trunk

Femoral n.

Obturator n.

Accessory Obturator n.

Sacral (Posterior Division)

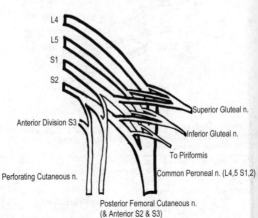

L4
L5
S1
S2

Superior Gluteal n.

Anterior Division S3

Inferior Gluteal n.

To Piriformis

Perforating Cutaneous n.

Common Peroneal n. (L4,5 S1,2)

Posterior Femoral Cutaneous n.
(& Anterior S2 & S3)

Sacral (Anterior Division)

L4
L5
S1
S2
S3
S4

To Quadratus Femoris & Inferior Gemellus

Pudendal

Posterior Femoral Cutaneous n. (& Posterior S1 & S2)

Tibial n. (L4,5 S1,2,3)

To Obturator Internus & Superior Gemellus

Dermatomes

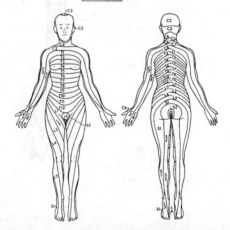

PERIPHERAL NERVES MOTOR INNERVATION

Axillary (C5,6) and Musculocutaneous (C[4],5,6,7)

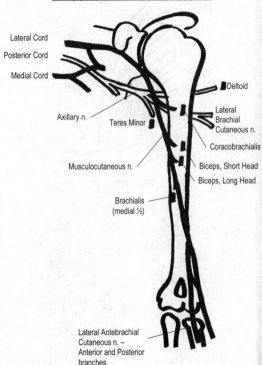

Lateral Cord

Posterior Cord

Medial Cord

Deltoid

Axillary n.

Teres Minor

Lateral Brachial Cutaneous n.

Coracobrachialis

Musculocutaneous n.

Biceps, Short Head

Biceps, Long Head

Brachialis (medial ½)

Lateral Antebrachial Cutaneous n. – Anterior and Posterior branches

Median (C[5],6,7,8 T1)

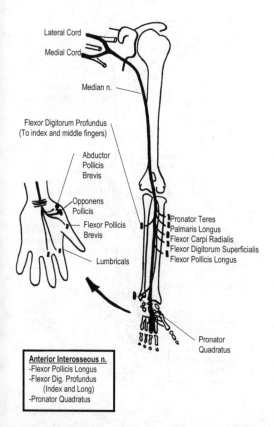

Lateral Cord
Medial Cord

Median n.

Flexor Digitorum Profundus
(To index and middle fingers)

Abductor
Pollicis
Brevis

Opponens
Pollicis

Flexor Pollicis
Brevis

Lumbricals

Pronator Teres
Palmaris Longus
Flexor Carpi Radialis
Flexor Digitorum Superficialis
Flexor Pollicis Longus

Pronator
Quadratus

Anterior Interosseous n.
-Flexor Pollicis Longus
-Flexor Dig. Profundus
  (Index and Long)
-Pronator Quadratus

Radial (C5,6,7,8 T1)

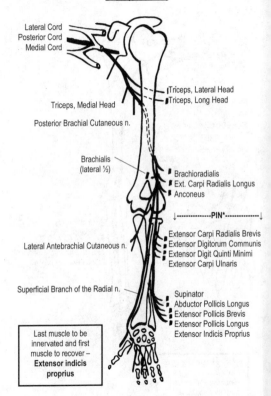

Lateral Cord
Posterior Cord
Medial Cord

Triceps, Lateral Head
Triceps, Long Head

Triceps, Medial Head

Posterior Brachial Cutaneous n.

Brachialis
(lateral ½)

Brachioradialis
Ext. Carpi Radialis Longus
Anconeus

↓-------------- PIN* --------------↓

Extensor Carpi Radialis Brevis
Extensor Digitorum Communis
Extensor Digit Quinti Minimi
Extensor Carpi Ulnaris

Lateral Antebrachial Cutaneous n.

Superficial Branch of the Radial n.

Supinator
Abductor Pollicis Longus
Extensor Pollicis Brevis
Extensor Pollicis Longus
Extensor Indicis Proprius

Last muscle to be
innervated and first
muscle to recover –
**Extensor indicis
proprius**

*PIN = Posterior interosseous nerve

Ulnar (C[7],8 T1)

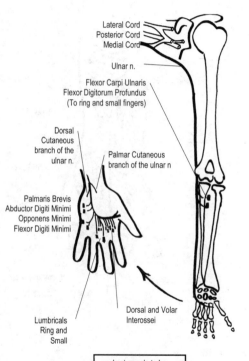

Lateral Cord
Posterior Cord
Medial Cord

Ulnar n.

Flexor Carpi Ulnaris
Flexor Digitorum Profundus
(To ring and small fingers)

Dorsal
Cutaneous
branch of the
ulnar n.

Palmar Cutaneous
branch of the ulnar n

Palmaris Brevis
Abductor Digiti Minimi
Opponens Minimi
Flexor Digiti Minimi

Lumbricals
Ring and
Small

Dorsal and Volar
Interossei

Last muscle to be
innervated –
1st Dorsal Interosseous

<u>Femoral (L2,3,4 [posterior]) and Obturator (L2,3,4 [anterior])</u>

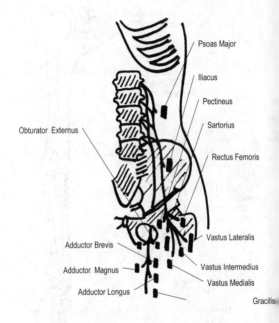

Superior Gluteal –
   Gluteus Medius and Minimus, Tensor Fascia Lata
Inferior Gluteal –
   Gluteus Maximus

Sciatic - Tibial Division (L4,5 S1,2,3)

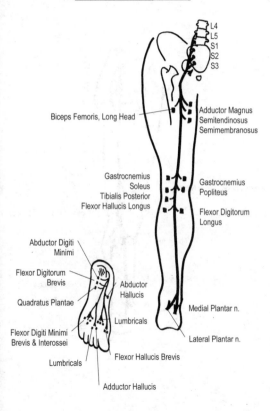

L4
L5
S1
S2
S3

Biceps Femoris, Long Head

Adductor Magnus
Semitendinosus
Semimembranosus

Gastrocnemius
Soleus
Tibialis Posterior
Flexor Hallucis Longus

Gastrocnemius
Popliteus

Flexor Digitorum
Longus

Abductor Digiti
Minimi

Flexor Digitorum
Brevis

Abductor
Hallucis

Quadratus Plantae

Lumbricals

Flexor Digiti Minimi
Brevis & Interossei

Medial Plantar n.

Lateral Plantar n.

Lumbricals

Flexor Hallucis Brevis

Adductor Hallucis

Sciatic - Common Peroneal Division (L4,5 S1,2)

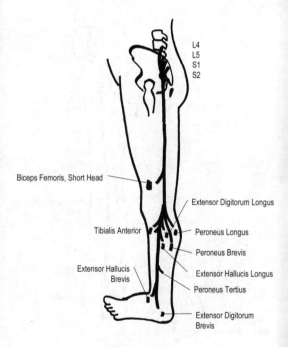

L4
L5
S1
S2

Biceps Femoris, Short Head

Extensor Digitorum Longus

Tibialis Anterior

Peroneus Longus

Peroneus Brevis

Extensor Hallucis
Brevis

Extensor Hallucis Longus

Peroneus Tertius

Extensor Digitorum
Brevis

PERIPHERAL NERVE SENSORY INNERVATION

<u>Anterior</u>   <u>Posterior</u>

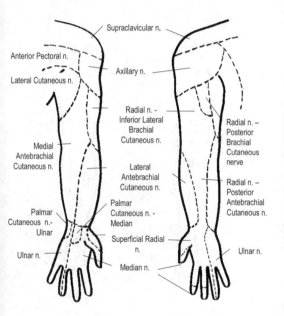

Supraclavicular n.

Anterior Pectoral n.

Axillary n.

Lateral Cutaneous n.

Radial n. - Inferior Lateral Brachial Cutaneous n.

Radial n. – Posterior Brachial Cutaneous nerve

Medial Antebrachial Cutaneous n.

Lateral Antebrachial Cutaneous n.

Radial n. – Posterior Antebrachial Cutaneous n.

Palmar Cutaneous n.- Ulnar

Palmar Cutaneous n. - Median

Ulnar n.

Superficial Radial n.

Ulnar n.

Median n.

<u>Anterior</u>   <u>Posterior</u>

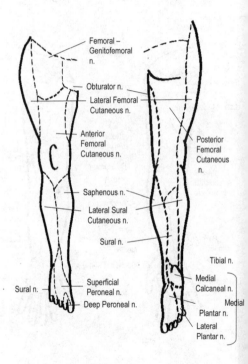

Femoral – Genitofemoral n.

Obturator n.

Lateral Femoral Cutaneous n.

Anterior Femoral Cutaneous n.

Posterior Femoral Cutaneous n.

Saphenous n.

Lateral Sural Cutaneous n.

Sural n.

Tibial n.

Sural n.

Superficial Peroneal n.

Deep Peroneal n.

Medial Calcaneal n.

Medial Plantar n.

Lateral Plantar n.

PERIPHERAL DERMATOMES

Upper Extremity

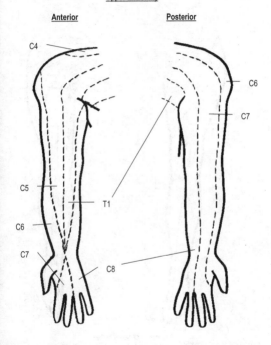

Lower Extremity

Anterior   **Posterior**

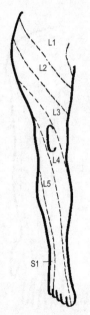
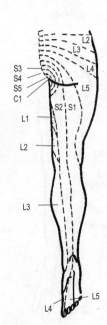

References for Anatomy Section
Hollingshead, W.H.: Anatomy for Surgeons, vol. 3, 2nd ed. NY, Harper and Rowe, 1969.
Hoppenfeld, S., and DeBoer, P. Surgical Exposures in Orthopaedics: The Anatomic Approach. 2 ed.
Philadelphia, J.B. Lippincott, 1994.
Miller, MD. (ed.) Review of Orthopaedics, 3rd ed. Philadelphia, W.B. Saunders, 2000.
Netter, F.H. The CIBA Collection of Medical Illustrations, Vol. 8. NJ. CIBA-Geigy Corp. 1991.
Pansky, B. Review of Gross Anatomy, 5th ed. NY. Macmillin Pub. Co.,1984.

Arthritis – Septic

Typically requires operative drainage and antibiotics. Empiric therapy is initiated following cultures (blood, synovial fluid)

Acute Single Joint

Age/Condition	Common Microbes	Treatment/Notes
Birth - 3 months	S. aureus, Enterobacter, Group B streptococcus, N. gonorrhea	1st: Penicillinase resistant synthetic PCN & 3rd generation cephalosporin 2nd: Penicillinase resistant synthetic PCN or vancomycin (MRSA) & anti pseudomonal aminoglycoside Note: Also consider contiguous osteomyelitis. Especially in femoral head, proximal humerus, and radial head (up to 60% positive)
3 months - 14 years	S. aureus, S. pyogenes, S. pneumonia, H. influenza, gram negative bacilli	1st: Penicillinase resistant synthetic PCN & 3rd generation cephalosporin 2nd: vancomycin & 3rd generation cephalosporin
15 - 40 years (sexually active)	N. gonorrhea, S. aureus, Streptococcus, rare aerobic gram negative bacilli	1st: gram stain negative = ceftriaxone 1g IV QD or cefotaxime or ceftizoxime 1g IV q8h 2nd: gram positive cocci in clusters = nafcillin or oxacillin 2 g IV q4h Note: S. aureus accounts for 50 - 80%. Cultures usually blood negative, joint positive. N. gonorrhea may not require operative irrigation and debridement.
> 40 years, positive rheumatoid (Rh)	S. aureus, Streptococcus, gram negative bacilli	1st: Penicillinase resistant synthetic PCN & 3rd generation cephalosporin 2nd: Penicillinase resistant synthetic PCN & ciprofloxacin Note: Consider CPPD & gout (See Joint fluid analysis section)
> 40 years, negative Rh	N. gonorrhea, S. aureus	1st: Penicillinase resistant synthetic PCN & 3rd generation cephalosporin 2nd: Penicillinase resistant synthetic PCN & ciprofloxacin
Total joint	S. aureus, epidermidis 20 - 30% Streptococcus, gram negative 15 - 25%, Anaerobic 5 - 10%	≤ 4-6 weeks: Irrigate & debride, antibiotics, retain prosthesis, 20-30% success >4-6 weeks: Irrigate & debride, removal of prosthesis, antibiotic spacer, IV antibiotics, reimplant 6 - 12 weeks (low virulence) 1 year (virulent), 90 - 95% success

Acute Multiple Joints

Age/Condition	Common Microbes	Treatment/Notes
Adult	N. gonorrhea, B. burgdorferi, Acute rheumatic fever, Hepatitis B, Parvovirus B19, Rubella vaccine	**1st:** ceftriaxone 1 g IV QD Gram stain not usually helpful! Remember to screen for sexually transmitted disease, Consider Lyme if indicated

Bites **No Pharmacological treatment substitutes for an adequate irrigation and if indicated a debridement of devitalized tissue.**

Age/Condition	Common Microbes	Treatment/Notes
Dog	V. streptococcus, P. multocida, S. aureus, E. corrodens, Bacteroides, Fusobacterium, Capnocytophaga canimonis (DF2), anaerobes	**1st:** amoxicillin/clavulanate (po) 875/125 mg BID or 500/125 mg TID **2nd:** clindamycin 300 mg QID & either fluoroquinoline (adults) or trimethoprim/ sulfamethoxazole (kids) **Note:** 5% of dog bites get infected, consider rabies
Cat	P. multocida, S. aureus	**1st:** amoxicillin/clavulanate (po) 875/125 mg BID or 500/125 mg TID **2nd:** cefuroxime 500 mg po q12h or doxycycline 100 mg po BID (NO cephalexin) **Note:** Soft tissue rest, consider surgical drainage, hand is a common site. Beware puncture of teeth into tendon sheaths/joints.
Cat scratch disease	B. henselea	**1st:** ciprofloxacin, trimethoprim/sulfamethoxazole, amoxicillin/clavulanate, macrolides **Note:** Efficacy not established
Catfish barb	Toxins	**1st:** amoxicillin/clavulanate (po) 875/125 mg BID or 500/125 mg TID **Note:** Antibiotics for prophylaxis. Barbs may need to be excised. Beware tendon sheath and joint penetration.
Miscellaneous -bat, raccoon, skunk, rat, pig	Poly-microbial, Streptobacillus monoliformis (rat)	**1st:** amoxicillin/clavulanate (po) 875/125 mg BID or 500/125 mg TID **2nd:** doxycycline 100 mg po BID (pig), 3rd generation cephalosporin, ticarcillin/ clavulanate, ampicillin/sulbactam, imipenum **Note:** Consider rabies immune globulin and vaccine if animal not available for testing or test positive.

Bites **No Pharmacological treatment substitutes for an adequate irrigation and if indicated a debridement of devitalized tissue.

Age/Condition	Common Microbes	Treatment/Notes
Human	S. aureus, E. corrodens, Streptococcus, anaerobes	1st: No infection: amoxicillin/clavulanate (po) 875/125 mg BID x 5d; Otherwise: ampicillin/sulbactam 1.5 g IV q6h or cefoxitin 2 g IV q8h or ticarcillin/clavulanate 3.1 g IV q6h or piperacillin/tazobactam 3.375 g IV q6h; PCN allergy: clindamycin & ciprofloxacin or trimethoprim/sulfamethoxazole **Note:** fight bites!! Unreliable history from intoxicated patient. Joint penetration = surgical drainage. Be sure to check location of wound in all degrees of joint range of motion. People punch with closed fists!!!
Snake (pit viper)	Pseudomonas, Enterobacter, S. epidermidis, Clostridium species	1st: Antibiotics as necessary prophylaxis with ceftriaxone **Note:** Anti-venom is treatment. Think tetanus! Follow for compartment syndrome.

Bursitis (May need wound debridement)

| Adult | S. aureus, rare Mycobacterium tuberculum & marinum | 1st: Penicillinase resistant synthetic PCN IV or po
2nd: 1st generation cephalosporin or vancomycin or ciprofloxacin
Note: Splint/soft tissue rest |

Diabetic Foot

| Previously treated, limited, no osteomyelitis | Aerobic gram positive cocci | 1st: clindamycin 300 mg po QID or 1st generation cephalosporin
Note: clindamycin 300 mg po QID or cephalexin 500 mg po QID x14d   90% cure |
| Chronic, recurrent limb threatening | Poly-microbial | 1st: Early: cefoxime or ciprofloxacin and (clindamycin or metronidazole)
2nd: Septic/Severe: imipenum or meropenum or ticarcillin/clavulanate or ampicillin/sulbactam or trovafloxacin or piperacillin/tazobactam or penicillinase resistant PCN & anti pseudomonal aminoglycoside or aztreonam and clindamycin
Note: Superficial ulcer cultures unreliable. Surgical debridement essential. High index of suspicion for necrotizing fasciitis or osteomyelitis. |

Hand/Paronychia

Age/Condition	Common Microbes	Treatment/Notes
Nail biting	S. aureus, anaerobes	**1st:** clindamycin 300 mg po QID **2nd:** erythromycin 500 mg po QID
Herpetic Whitlow	Herpes simplex	**1st:** acyclovir 400 mg po TID x 10 days **Notes:** Gram stain and culture negative. May be confused for a felon!
Water immersion	Candida species	**1st:** Topical clotrimazole **Note:** Avoid hand immersion

Osteomyelitis: A specific microbe diagnosis essential via blood and tissue cultures. The following represents the initial **empiric** treatment.

Age/Condition	Common Microbes	Treatment/Notes
0 – 4 months	S. aureus, gram negative bacilli, Group B streptococcus	**1st:** 3rd generation cephalosporin and either nafcillin or oxacillin **2nd:** vancomycin & 3rd generation cephalosporin **Note:** Look for local signs/symptoms. Blood culture often positive.
Children < 4 years	S. aureus, group A streptococcus	**1st:** nafcillin or oxacillin, gram negative add 3rd generation cephalosporin **2nd:** vancomycin or clindamycin **Note:** H. influenza in unimmunized. Vancomycin for PCN Allergic
Adult > 21 years	S. aureus most common	**1st:** nafcillin or oxacillin 2 g q4h IV or Ancef 2 g q8h IV **2nd:** vancomycin 1 g q12h IV **Note:** Tailor to culture results
Sickle cell anemia	S. aureus most common, consider Salmonella	**1st:** fluoroquinoline (adult) **2nd:** 3rd generation cephalosporin
Intravenous drug user	S. aureus, Pseudomonas	**1st:** Penicillinase resistant PCN & ciprofloxacin **2nd:** vancomycin & ciprofloxacin **Note:** Sternoclavicular joints, ribs, spine, long bones
Dialysis	S. aureus, Pseudomonas	**1st:** Penicillinase resistant PCN & ciprofloxacin **2nd:** vancomycin & ciprofloxacin

Osteomyelitis (Continued)

Age/Condition	Common Microbes	Treatment/Notes
After open reduction internal fixation (ORIF)	Coliforms, S. aureus, Pseudomonas	1st: nafcillin 2 g IV q4h and ciprofloxacin 750 mg po BID 2nd: vancomycin 1 g q12h IV and 3rd generation cephalosporin **Note:** Think of in nonunions and delayed unions
Sneaker puncture	Pseudomonas	1st: ceftazidime 2 g q8h IV or cefipime 2 g q12h IV 2nd: ciprofloxacin 750 mg po BID (adults) **Note:** Look for foreign body debride if necessary
Vascular insufficiency	Polymicrobial	1st: outpatient – amoxicillin/clavulanate 500 mg TID po 2nd: Inpatient - imipenum, meropenum, piperacillin/tazobactam, ampicillin /sulbactam, trovafloxacin, cefipime & metronidazole, or vancomycin & aztreonam & metronidazole **Note:** Total contact casting. Surgery for exposed bone or osteomyelitis
Chronic osteomyelitis	S. aureus, pseudomonas Enterobacter	Based on results of culture
Skin Infections		
Cellulitis - mild	Group A streptococcus, S. aureus	1st: dicloxacillin 500 mg po q6h or cefazolin 1 g q8h IV **Note:** Splint/soft tissue rest
Cellulitis - severe	Group A streptococcus, S. aureus	1st: nafcillin or oxacillin 2 g q4h IV 2nd: erythromycin or amoxicillin/clavulanate or azithromycin or clarithromycin or 1st generation cephalosporin **Note:** Irrigation & debridement of abscess

Infection Imitators: Gout/Pseudogout (polarized light microscopy), Calcific tendonitis (normal labs, intratendinous Mineralization), or Pyoderma gangrenosum

Skin Infections

Age/Condition	Common Microbes	Treatment/Notes
Infection – wound, severe	Polymicrobial: S. aureus, group A & anaerobic streptococcus, Enterobacter, C. perfringens & tetani, Pseudomonas, Aeromonas (water exposure)	1st: amoxicillin/clavulanate (po) 875/125 mg BID, 500/125 mg TID, or 1st generation cephalosporin Sepsis: ampicillin/sulbactam, ticarcillin/clavulanate, piperacillin/tazobactam, imipenum, or meropenum 2nd: erythromycin or clindamycin or azithromycin or clarithromycin Sepsis: ciprofloxacin, clindamycin and either nafcillin or oxacillin 2g IV q4h Note: Surgical debridement if needed, splint for soft tissue rest. Tailor antibiotic to cultured bug.
Necrotizing fasciitis	Streptococcus groups A, C, & G, Clostridia species, anaerobic & aerobic (polymicrobial)	Based on intraoperative gram stain and culture. Note: Wide Immediate Surgical Debridement: Soft tissue crepitance (gas in the subcutaneous tissue) may be the only early sign
Post-op infection	S. aureus, Group A streptococcus, Enterobacter	1st: cefoxitin, cefotetan, ticarcillin/clavulanate, piperacillin/tazobactam, ampicillin/sulbactam, or 2nd generation cephalosporin and either metronidazole or imipenum or meropenum Note: Early irrigation and debridement as indicated
Flexor tenosynovitis	S. aureus, Streptococcus, gram negative rods	1st: cefazolin 1 g IV q8h 2nd: nafcillin 1 - 2 g IV q4-6h, vancomycin 1 g IV q12h and gentamicin or imipenum 0.5 - 1 g IV q6h Note: IV antibiotics and observation if caught early (< 24 HOURS); maintain a low threshold for irrigation and debridement

Key Atypical Infections

Organism	Chemotherapy
Sporothrix scheckii	Ketoconazole, supersaturated solution of potassium iodide, amphotericin, surgical debridement
M. marinum	Rifampin, tetracycline, minocycline, amikacin
M. tuberculosis	Isoniazid, rifampin, ethambutol, pyrazinamide
M. avium	Azithromycin, clarithromycin, ethambutol, rifabutin

Common Antibiotics Mechanisms of Action

Inhibits	Antibiotics
Cell wall synthesis	Carbenicillin, cephalosporins, methicillin, nafcillin, oxacillin, penicillin, piperacillin, ticarcillin
Cell membrane function	Amphotericin, nystatin, polymyxin
Protein synthesis	Aminoglycosides, chloramphenicol, clindamycin, erythromycin, tetracycline
Nucleic acid synthesis	Sulfonamides
DNA gyrase	Quinolones
Bacterial RNA synthesis	Rifampin

Antibiotic References[3,4,5,6,7,8,9,10]

[3] The Harriet Lane Handbook 15th ed., St. Louis, Mosby Year Book. 1999.

[4] Browner BD, et. al. Skeletal Trauma. Philadelphia, WB Saunders. 1998.

[5] Gilbert DN, et. al. The Sanford Guide to Antimicrobial Therapy, VA Antimicrobial Therapy, Inc. 2000.

[6] Miller, MD. Review of Orthopaedics, 3rd ed. Philadelphia, WB Saunders. 2000.

[7] Bartlett JG. 1999 Pocket Book of Infectious Disease Therapy. Baltimore, William and Wilkins. 1998.

[8] Abrams RA, et. al. Hand Infections: Treatment Recommendations for specific types. JAAOS 1996;4:219-230.

[9] Neviaser, RJ. Acute Infections in Green's Operative Hand Surgery, 4th ed. Philadelphia, Churchill Livingstone, 1999.

[10] Patel MR. Chronic Infections in Green's Operative Hand Surgery, 4th ed. Philadelphia, Churchill Livingstone, 1999.

Common Pediatric Oral Antimicrobial Doses and Mixtures

Antimicrobial	Formulations	Dose (Frequency)
amoxicillin (Amoxil)	Suspension: 125, 250 mg/5ml, Capsules: 125, 250 mg	30-50 mg/kg/day (tid), Max dose 500 mg
amoxicillin/clavulanate (Augmentin)	Suspension: 200 & 400 mg/5ml, Tablets: 250, 500 mg	45 mg/kg/day (bid), Max dose 500 mg
ampicillin (Polycillin)	Suspension: 125, 250 mg/5ml, Capsules: 250, 500 mg	50-100 mg/kg/day (qid), Max dose 500 mg
azithromycin (Zithromax)	Suspension: 125, 1000 mg/5ml, Capsules: 250 mg, 1000 mg	10 mg/kg qd on 1st day, then 5 mg/kg qd x 4d Max dose 500 mg
cefaclor (Ceclor), 2nd generation	Suspension: 125, 250 mg/5ml, Capsules: 250, 500 mg	20 – 40 mg/kg/day (tid), Max dose 500 mg
cefadroxil (Duricef), 1st generation	Suspension: 125,250,500 mg/5ml, Capsules: 500, Tab: 1000 mg	30 mg/kg/day (bid), Max dose 1000 mg
cefixime (Suprax), 3rd generation	Syrup: 100 mg/5ml, Tablets: 200, 400 mg	8 mg/kg/day (qd/bid), Max dose 400 mg
cefpodoxime (Vantin), 3rd generation	Suspension: 50, 100 mg/5ml, Tablets: 100, 200 mg	10 mg/kg/day (bid), Max dose 400 mg
cefprozil (Cefzil), 3rd generation	Suspension: 125, 250 mg/5ml, Tablets: 250 mg/5ml	15 mg/kg/day (bid), Max dose 500 mg
ceftibuten (Cedax), 3rd generation	Suspension: 90, 180 mg/5ml, Capsules: 400 mg	9 mg/dg/day (qd), Max dose 400 mg
cefuroxime (Ceftin), 2nd generation	Suspension: 125 mg/5ml, Tablets: 125, 250, 500 mg	15 - 30 mg/kg/day (bid), Max dose 500 mg

Common Pediatric Oral Antimicrobial Doses and Mixtures (Continued)

Antimicrobial	Formulations	Dose (Frequency)
cephalexin (Keflex), 1st generation	Suspension: 125, 250 mg/5ml, Capsules: 250, 500 mg	25-50 mg/kg/day (qid), Max dose 500 mg
clarithromycin (Biaxin)	Suspension: 125, 250 mg/5 ml, Tablets: 250, 500 mg	15 mg/kg/day (bid), Max dose 500 mg
clindamycin (Cleocin)	Solution: 75 mg/5ml, Capsules: 75,150 mg	10 - 25 mg/kg/day (tid/bid), Max dose 600 mg
dicloxacillin (Dynapen)	Suspension: 62.5 mg/5ml, Capsules: 125, 250, 500	25 - 100 mg/kg/day (qid), Max dose 500 mg
erythromycin (ERYC, EES, E-mycin)	Suspension:200, 400 mg/5ml, Tablets: 200(chew),250,400,500	20 - 50 mg/kg/day (qid), Max dose 500 mg
erythromycin/sulfisoxazole (Pediazole)	Suspension: 200 mg erythromycin & 600 mg sulfisoxazole per 5ml	50 mg erythromycin/kg/day (qid), Max erythromycin dose 500 mg
loracarbef (Lorabid), 2nd generation	Suspension: 100, 200 mg/5ml, Capsules: 200 mg	15 - 30 mg/kg/day (bid), Max dose 400 mg
penicillin (Pen-Vee K)	Suspension: 125, 250, Tablets: 125, 250, 500 mg	25 - 50 mg/kg/day (qid), Max dose 500 mg
trimethoprim / sulfamethoxazole (Bactrim, Septra)	Suspension: 40 mg trimethoprim & 200 mg Sulfamethoxazole per 5ml Tablets: 80/400, 160/800	6-12 mg trimethoprim & 30 – 60 mg sulfamethoxazole per kg/day (bid), Max dose 160 mg trimethoprim

Modified with permission from *Tarascon Pediatric Emergency Pocketbook*, 3rd ed., Tarascon Publishing, Loma Linda, CA

Emergency Procedures

Compartment Syndrome[11]

Pressure increase may be intrinsic
-Bleeding, Edema, Fluid

> Increased pressure within a confined space interferes with proper circulation within the space.

Or extrinsic
-Pneumatic anti shock trousers,
Cast, Tight dressing

Findings

-Pain out of proportion to physical findings (**_pain is the most reliable and earliest sign_**), Pain with passive ROM, pain on palpation of the swollen compartment, tensely swollen compartment, tight shiny skin, hypesthesia, paraesthesia, anesthesia (late finding), weakness, paresis (late finding). Late findings occur after irreversible damage has occurred!

Compartment Pressure Values[12,13]

Compartment syndrome is felt to be present if compartment pressures are:	Within 10 –30 mm Hg of diastolic pressure
	OR
	Above 45 mm Hg – absolute pressure

Needle manometer measurements are generally allowed to be slightly higher. Most surgeons prefer to use the measurement of compartment pressure relative to diastolic pressure. A "zone of peak pressure" occurs within several cm of the fracture site; values can vary significantly at greater distances causing an underestimation of the compartment pressure.

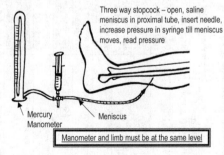

Three way stopcock – open, saline meniscus in proximal tube, insert needle, increase pressure in syringe till meniscus moves, read pressure

Mercury Manometer   Meniscus

> **Manometer and limb must be at the same level**

[11] Whitesides TE, Heckman MM. Acute Compartment Syndrome: Update on diagnosis and treatment. JAAOS 1996;4:209-218.

[12] Mcqueen, MM., Court-Brown, CM.: Compartment Monitoring in Tibial Fractures. JBJS 78B:99-104, 1996.

[13] Matsen, FA. et. al.: Diagnosis and Management of Compartment Syndromes. JBJS 62A:286-291, 1980.

Measuring Techniques (multiple)

Needle Manometer[14], Wick catheter[15], Slit catheter [16], Stic catheter

The simplest technique utilizes the Stic Catheter. It is a handheld device made by Stryker that is easy to use and usually readily available at larger institutions. Another simple technique is to use an arterial line set-up. This can be connected to a standard pressure monitor at the bedside or in the OR. Additionally, the arterial line set up comes in a sterile package and can then be used intraoperatively with the help of the OR nurse or anesthetist. Ensure the set-up is "zero'd" at the level of the limb being tested.

Compartment Release (Fasciotomy) Techniques

Finger[17]

Usually done on the ulnar side of the index, long, and ring fingers and the radial side of the thumb and small finger. Special attention and alteration of this should be based on the patient's vocation and avocation. The incision is a standard mid-axial incision as shown. The line for the mid-axial incision is drawn off points that correspond to the dorsal extent of the flexion creases in maximal flexion. The volar neurovascular bundles are left volar and the line of dissection is between them and the flexor tendon sheath.

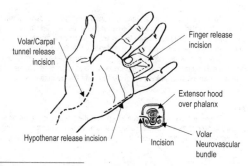

Volar/Carpal tunnel release incision

Finger release incision

Extensor hood over phalanx

Hypothenar release incision

Incision

Volar Neurovascular bundle

---

[14] Whitesides, TE., et. al.: Tissue Pressure Measurement as a determinant for the need of Fasciotomy. Clin Orthop 1975;113:43.

[15] Mubarak, SJ., Hargens, AR., Owen, CA., et al: The Wick Catheter Technique for Measurement of Intramuscular Pressure: A New Research and Clinical Tool. JBJS 1976;58A:1016.

[16] Rorabek, CH., Castle GSP., Hardie, R., et al: Compartmental Pressure Measurements: An Experimental Investigation Using the Slit Catheter. J Trauma 1981;21:446-449.

[17] Green, DP (ed.) Operative Hand Surgery. NY. Churchill Livingstone, 1993.

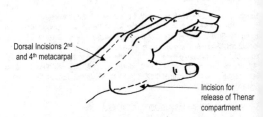

Dorsal Incisions 2nd
and 4th metacarpal

Incision for
release of Thenar
compartment

Hand

The volar incision lies in the crease between the thenar and hypothenar eminences. From it one can release the Carpal tunnel and Guyon's canal. The incision is curved over the wrist flexion crease to prevent contractures.

The dorsal incisions are made in line with the second and fourth metacarpals as shown. The incisions split the dorsal interossei fascia and then course around the muscle to release the palmar interossei. The thenar and hypothenar compartments are released through incisions over the respective metacarpals.

Forearm[18,19,20]

Two incisions one dorsal and one volar are used to decompress the forearm. The volar incision includes the carpal tunnel release. Taking the incision ulnar after the carpal tunnel release leaves tissue to cover the median nerve as it exits from under the Flexor digitorum superficialis. The dorsal incision should be used to decompress the dorsal and mobile wad compartments. Intraoperative pressure measurements can aid in making the decision to proceed with the dorsal release. Often the volar release is sufficient to lower the pressure dorsally to sub critical levels.

Arm

The volar incision can be carried up past the elbow and into an anterior lateral approach to the arm to release brachial compartments if necessary. Anterior and posterior compartments may then be released through the anterolateral incision.

---

[18] Gelberman, et. al. Decompression of Compartment Syndromes of the Forearm. Clin Orthop. 1978;134:225-229.

[19] Gelberman, et. al. Compression syndromes of the Forearm Diagnosis and Treatment. Clin Orthop. 1981;161:252-261.

[20] Green, DP (ed.) Surgery of the Hand. Phila. Lippincott, 1990.

Forearm release incisions

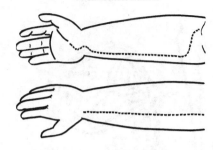

Thigh[21]

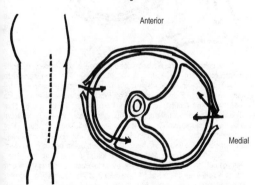

Thigh compartment syndromes are being more commonly reported. The incisions are anterolateral and if needed straight medial. The hamstring compartment is released via the anterolateral incision.

---

[21] Tarlow SD. et al. Acute Compartment Syndrome in the Thigh Complicating Fracture of the Femur. JBJS 1986;68A:1439.

Leg[22]

Anterior

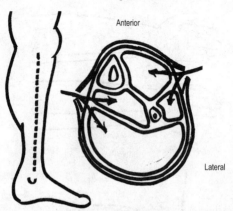

Lateral

Three common techniques for fasciotomy of the leg exist; fibulectomy, peri-fibular fasciotomy, and the double incision technique. The most commonly advocated is the double incision technique. The two vertical incisions must be separated by at least a 8 cm skin bridge. Both incisions span from knee to ankle. The medial incision is at least 2 cm posterior to the posteromedial border of the tibia (avoids bone exposure and damage to the Saphenous nerve and vein). The fascia overlying the gastrocnemius is split to release the superficial compartment. The deep compartment fascia is split over the flexor digitorum longus and proximally the soleal attachment to the tibia is released to access the proximal portion of the deep posterior compartment (Tibialis posterior). The lateral incision is made midway between the posterolateral tibial border and the anterolateral border of the fibula. The fascia is split 1 cm anterior and 1 cm posterior to the intramuscular septum. The superficial peroneal nerve must be protected.

---
[22] Mubarak, SJ., Owen, CA.: Double-Incision Fasciotomy of the Leg for Decompression in Compartment Syndromes. JBJS 59A:184-187, 1977.

Foot[23],[24]

A foot compartment syndrome is difficult to detect. Clinical suspicion and pressure measurement are necessary to identify those requiring release. Two techniques are shown below. The main compartments are medial, central, lateral, interosseous, and calcaneal. All involved compartments should be released if indicated.

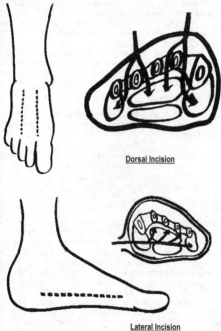

Dorsal Incision

Lateral Incision

[23] Takhouri, AJ. Manoli AII. Acute foot compartment syndromes. J. Orthop. Trauma. 1992;223-228.
[24] Myerson, MS. Diagnosis and Treatment of Compartment Syndromes of the Foot. Orthopedics 1990;13:711-717.

Important to note![25]

There is universal agreement that acute compartment syndromes should be treated surgically. However, the treatment of compartment syndromes presenting late with evidence of compartment damage is less clear. The damage done in a compartment is a function of many variables including; compartment pressure magnitude, time of pressure elevation, diastolic pressure, concomitant crush injury, and time since onset among others. It has been shown that late release of compartments is associated with an unacceptable complication rate. Hard and fast rules regarding the treatment of compartment syndromes do not exist. The guidelines given above along with heightened clinical suspicion and an educated response are most appropriate.

Ensure you check serum CPK's and place a Foley catheter to monitor urine color. If positive for myoglobinuria, treat with aggressive hydration and alkalinization with sodium bicarbonate. **A urine dipstick positive for blood in the absence of RBC's on microscopic analysis is indicative of myoglobinuria.

Acute Stabilization of the Pelvis

Hemodynamic instability in the presence of a grossly negative DPL (or other negative abdominal imaging study) and an unstable pelvis is an indication for acute pelvic stabilization.

Methods

Pneumatic anti shock garment including abdominal compartment (Has been associated with compartment syndromes/subsequent amputation)	
Blanket wrapped around the pelvis and clamped snuggly	
Internal rotation of the legs and wrapping both together	
Skeletal traction	Pelvic binder
Specialized pelvic clamps[26]	Anterior external fixation frame

Use 5 mm pins with the threads placed in the anterior half of the iliac crest. Pins must be at least 1 cm apart. 2 - 3 pins per side. Stab incisions are made along the crest and angled towards the umbilicus. The crest is identified and the walls may be palpated and/or the proper angle of the crest identified with a guide wire. The crest is perforated with a drill; the pin is then inserted and allowed to find its way between the inner and outer table. All pins should be directed towards the strong bone in the supra-acetabular region. All threads should be buried in the crest bone. Pin placement is confirmed after reduction and prior to leaving the OR.

Frame construction should take into consideration possible need for abdominal exploration, interventional venous thrombosis, and concomitant injuries. Double frame can be helpful to allow access to belly without loss of fixation.

[25] Finkelstein, JA, Hunter, GA., Hu, RW.: Lower limb compartment syndrome: Course after delayed fasciotomy. J Trauma 1996;40(3):342-344.

[26] Buckle, R., Browner, BD., Morandi, M. A new external fixation device for emergent reduction and stabilization of displaced pelvic fractures associated with massive hemorrhage. J Orthop Trauma 1993;7:177-178.

Regulation of Calcium and Phosphate Metabolism[27,28]

Parameter	Parathyroid Hormone (PTH)	1,25-(OH)$_2$ Vitamin D	Calcitonin
Origin	Parathyroid chief cells	Kidney proximal tubules	Thyroid parafollicular cells
Factors that stimulate production	↓ Serum Calcium	↑ PTH ↓ Serum Calcium ↓ Serum Phosphorus	↑ Serum Calcium
Factors that inhibit production	↑ Serum Calcium ↑ 1,25-(OH)$_2$ D	↓ PTH ↑ Serum Calcium ↑ Serum Phosphorus	↓ Serum Calcium
Effect on end organ			
Intestine	No direct effect Acts indirectly on bowel by ↑ 1,25-(OH)$_2$ D in Kidney	↑↑ Intestinal uptake of Calcium and Phosphorous	?
Kidney	↑ 25-(OH) D to 1,25-(OH)$_2$ D in proximal tubules ↑ resorption of filtered Calcium ↑ urinary loss of Phosphorus	?	?
Bone	↑ osteoclastic activity ↑ pre osteoclasts	↑↑ osteoclastic activity	↓ osteoclastic activity
Net effect on Ca+ and phosphorous (serum and extra cellular fluid)	↑ Serum Calcium ↓ Serum phosphorus	↑ Serum Calcium ↑ Serum Phosphorus	Transient ↓ Serum Calcium

Adapted from Miller MD (ed): Review of Orthopaedics, 3rd ed. Philadelphia, WB Saunders, 2000, page 23, with permission

27 Mankin HJ. Metabolic Bone Disease. JBJS 77A:459-469, 1995
28 Brinker, MR. Basic Sciences. In Review of Orthopaedics,3rd ed. Pp 1-144. Philadelphia, PA, WB Saunders, 2000.

Clinical and Radiologic Overview of Metabolic Bone Disease

Disease	Etiology	Clinical Findings	Radiographic Finding
Hypercalcemia			
Hyperparathyroid	↑ PTH - adenoma	Kidney stones, hyperreflexia	Osteopenia, osteitis fibrosa cystica
Familial syndromes	↑ PTH – MEN/Renal	Endocrine/renal dysfunction	Osteopenia
Hypocalcemia			
Hypoparathyroidism	↓ PTH – idiopathic	Neuromuscular irritability, eye	Calcified basal ganglia
PHP/Albright's	PTH receptor dysfunction	Short metacarpal/tarsal Obesity	Brachydactyly, exostosis
Renal osteodystrophy	CRF – ↓ phosphate excretion	Renal abnormalities	"Rugger jersey" spine
Rickets (osteomalacia)			
Vit. D deficient	↓ Diet vitamin D, malabsorption	Osteomalacia, hypotonia, muscle weakness, tetany.	Rachitic rosary, bowed long bones, ↑ growth plates
Vit. D dependent (Types I & II)	I enzyme defect, II receptor defect	Similar but ↑ (I) to ↑↑ (II) severity to vitamin D dependent, alopecia	Poor mineralization
Vit. D resistant (hypophosphatemic)	↓ phosphate resorption (tubular)	Hypophosphatemia, Lower limb deformities, stunted growth	Poor mineralization
Hypophosphatasia	↓ Alkaline phosphatase	Osteomalacia, early tooth loss	Poor mineralization
Osteopenia			
Osteoporosis	↓ estrogen → ↓ bone mass	Kyphosis, fracture	Insufficiency fractures
Scurvey	↓ Diet Vitamin C	Fatigue, bleeding, effusions	Thin cortices, corner sign
Osteodense			
Paget's (5th decade)	Defunct osteoclasts, disordered bone turnover	Deformity, pain, congestive heart failure, fractures	Coarse thick trabeculae, Picture frame vertebrae
Osteopetrosis	Osteo/chondroclastic activity(thymus)	Hepatosplenomegaly, anemia	Bone within bone

MEN multiple endocrine neoplasia, PTH Parathyroid hormone, PHP Pseudo hypoparathyroidism
CRF Chronic renal failure,
Adapted from Miller MD (ed): Review of Orthopaedics, 3rd ed. Philadelphia, WB Saunders, 2000, page 25 with permission

OSTEOPOROSIS[29,30]

Type I (postmenopausal)
Type II Age related (> 75 years old)
   Affects 45% of women > 50 years old
   Lifetime risk of 40% for fractures
   Treatment may reduce risk by 50%
   Normal Laboratory values

> **DEXA (Osteoporosis criteria)**
> Based on 25 year old control
> T-score
> -2.0 SD without risk factors
> -1.5 SD with risk factors
> DEXA study is the most accurate
> DEXA has the least radiation

Plain films reveal osteopenia > 30%

Calcium Recommendations

Age Range	RDA, mg/day	Suggested Dietary Intake, mg/day
Infants		
Birth – 3 months	400	400
6 – 12 months	600	600
Children		
1 - 5 years	800	800
5 - 10 years	800	800 - 1200
Adolescents/Adult		
11 - 24 years	1200	1200 - 1500
Female Athletes		
Euestrogenemic	Not specified	1000
Hypoestrogenemic	Not specified	1500
Adults		
Men (25 - 65)	800	1000
Women (25 - 55)	800	1500
Pregnant/Nursing	1200	1200 - 1500
Postmenopausal		
With HRT*	Not specified	1000
Without HRT*	Not specified	1500
> 65 Men/Women	800	1500

> **Osteoporosis risk factors**
> -Sedentary
> -Thin
> -Caucasian
> -N. European
> -Smoker
> -Alcohol
> -Phenytoin
> -Low calcium
> -Low vitamin D
> -Breast feeding
> -Any adult fracture

*HRT Hormone replacement therapy
Adapted from Subcommittee on the Tenth Edition of the Recommended Dietary Allowance, National Research Council: Recommended Daily Allowances, 10th ed. Washington, DC. National Academic Press, 1989.
Table adapted from Lane JM and Nydick M. Osteoporosis: Current Modes of Prevention and Treatment. JAAOS Jan/Feb 1999, p. 23.

[29] Lane JM and Nydick M. Osteoporosis: Current Modes of Prevention and Treatment. JAAOS 1999;7:19-31.
[30] Freedman KB, et al. Treatment of osteoporosis: Are physicians missing an opportunity? J Bone Joint Surg 2000;82-A:1063-1070.

Treatment Protocols[31]

<u>Men and Pre menopausal women</u>

  Physiologic Calcium, Vitamin D (400 – 800 U/day), Adequate nutrition, Exercise

<u>Post menopausal women*</u>

Antiresorptive agents

- Estrogens (consider progestin if uterus intact)
- alendronate (Fosamax), 5 mg/day for mild to moderate bone deficiency; 10 mg/day if bone mass 2.0 SD's below peak bone mass
- calcitonin (Miacalcin), 200 U/day via nasal spray for mild bone loss, new fractures, or bone pain
- pamidronate (Aredia; intravenous infusion), approved for Paget's disease and osteolysis associated with malignancy
- raloxifene (Evista), an anti estrogen (SERM) approved for prevention

Not approved by FDA (experimental)

- etidronate (Didronel), cycle of 400 mg/day for 2 weeks, rest 11 weeks; Approved for Paget's disease only
- tamoxifen (Nolvadex; antiestrogen agent), 70% as effective as estrogen, Used in the treatment of breast cancer

Formative agents (experimental)

- monofluorophosphate (Monocal; fluoride and calcium supplement), 24 mg of elemental fluoride per day, used as a nutritional additive
- Slow-release sodium fluoride, under study

*Earlier intervention if the bone loss rate is increased and/or there are independent risk factors

Osteonecrosis

Etiologies

-Alcoholism	-Antiphospholipid antibody syndrome
-Dysbaric disorders	-Endotoxic reactions/systemic bacterial infections
-Gaucher's disease	-Hyperlipidemia (Types II and IV)
-Hemiglobinopathies (HbS)	-Inflammatory (lupus, inflammatory bowel disease)
-Hypercoagulable states	-Trauma (dislocation, neck fracture)
-Irradiation	-Pregnancy
-Viral etiologies (hepatitis, HIV, CMV, rubella, rubeola, varicella	
-Hypersensitivity states (anaphylaxis, allograft rejection)	
-Malignancy (metastatic carcinoma, acute promyelocytic and lymphoid leukemia)	
-Hypercortisolism (endogenous [Cushing's] and exogenous)	

MRI – Single best study to detect Osteonecrosis 98% specificity

---

[31] Lane JM and Nydick M. Osteoporosis: Current Modes of Prevention and Treatment. JAAOS 1999, p. 23.

Staging System for Osteonecrosis of the Hip
Steinberg modification of the Ficat/Arlet classification[32]

Stage	Criteria
O	Normal radiographs, bone scan, and MRI
I	Normal radiographs, positive bone scan and/or MRI
II	Abnormal radiographs - cystic or sclerotic changes in femoral head
III	Abnormal radiographs - subchondral collapse/*crescent sign*
IV	Abnormal radiographs - femoral head flattening
V	Abnormal radiographs - loss of joint space +/- acetabular changes
VI	Abnormal radiographs - degenerative changes (advanced)

Stages are graded on the quantity of the femoral head involvement. Involvement is calculated by taking the product of the % involvement on the coronal AP and the sagittal lateral.

Stage	Grading	Criteria
II	A	< 20% head involvement on radiographs or MRI
	B	20 - 40%
	C	> 40%
III	A	Crescent (subchondral collapse) < 15%, no flattening
	B	15 - 30% crescent, no flattening
	C	> 30% crescent, no flattening
IV	A	< 15% collapse and < 2 mm depression
	B	15-30% or 2-4 mm
	C	> 30% or > 4 mm
V	A	Mild (IV & includes estimate of acetabular involvement)
	B	Moderate (IV & includes estimate of acetabular involvement)
	C	Severe (IV & includes estimate of acetabular involvement)

Natural History
Necrotic sector small (<15%) - May resolve, prognosis usually good
Necrotic sector large (> 50%) - Collapse and arthrosis 85%, usually needs a total hip replacement

Treatment Options (among others)
Observation (crutches, unload joint)
Core decompression
Vascularized fibular strut grafting
Rotational osteotomy
Hip arthrodesis
Hip arthroplasty

---

[32] Steinberg ME, Hayken GD, Steinberg DR. A quantitative system for staging avascular necrosis. J Bone Joint Surg 1995;77B:34.

Joint arthroplasty antibiotic prophylaxis dental procedure recommendations[33]

Potentially increased risk:	Consider prophylaxis for:
Immunocompromised/suppressed	(Higher incidence of bacteremia)
Rheumatoid arthritis	Extractions
Systemic lupus erythematosus	Periodontal procedures
Disease, drug, or radiation induced	Dental implants/replants
Other:	Endodontic (root canal) procedures
Insulin dependent diabetes	Placement of orthodontic bands
1st 2 years post arthroplasty	Intraligamentary anesthetic injection
Previous prosthetic joint infection	Cleaning where bleeding is expected
Malnourishment	
Hemophilia	

Modified with permission from Dajani, AS, et. al. Prevention of Bacterial Endocarditis: Recommendations by the American Heart Association. JAMA 1997;277(22):1794-1801. Copyrighted 1997 AMA.

Suggested antibiotic prophylaxis if criteria are met

PCN tolerant	amoxicillin, cephalexin, cephradine - 2 gm po 1 hour prior
PCN allergic	clindamycin - 600 mg po 1 hour prior
Can't take po, PCN tolerant	ampicillin - 2 gm IV/IM 1 hour prior OR cefazolin - 1 gm IV/IM 1 hour prior
Can't take po, PCN allergic	Clindamycin - 600 mg IV/IM 1 hour prior

Suggested antibiotic prophylaxis for GU/GI Procedures

PCN tolerant	Pre procedure	Post procedure
ampicillin & gentamicin	1.5 mg/kg (80 mg) IV 30 minutes prior	
amoxicillin		1.5 gm po 6 hours post
PCN allergic		
vancomycin & gentamicin	1 gm IV & 1.5 mg/kg IV (~80) 1 hour prior	Repeat 8 hours post

Wound Classification for tetanus prophylaxis

Clinical Features	Tetanus Prone	Non-Tetanus Prone
Age of wound	> 6 hours	≤6 hours
Configuration	Stellate, avulsion	Linear
Depth	> 1 cm	≤1 cm
Mechanism	Missile, crush, burn, frostbite	Sharp surface (glass, knife)
Devitalized Tissue	Present	Absent
Contaminants (dirt, saliva)	Present	Absent

[33] Antibiotic Prophylaxis for Dental Patients with Total Joint Replacements. JADA 1997;128(7):1004-8. Copyright © 1997 American Dental Association and American Academy of Orthopaedic Surgery. Adapted 2001 with permission of ADA publishing, a Division of ADA Business Enterprises, Inc.

Tetanus Immunization Schedule[b]

	Tetanus Prone		Non Tetanus Prone	
Tetanus Product	Td[c]	TIG	Td	TIG
Unknown, < 3 doses	Yes	Yes	Yes	No
3 or more doses	No[d]	No	No[e]	No

b – Data from Morbidity and Mortality Weekly Report 39:37, 1990., c – Yes if wound >24 hours old. For children < 7 yr., DPT (DT if Pertussis vaccine contraindicated) for persons ≥ 7 yr, Td preferred to tetanus toxoid alone, d – Yes if > 5 yr since last booster
e – Yes if > 10 yr since last booster

Joint Fluid Analysis[34]

Types	I - Non inflammatory	II - Inflammatory	III - Septic	IV - Hemorrhagic

Gross examination

Blood (hemarthrosis), Fat (violation of subchondral bone/fracture)
The more inflammatory a fluid is the more opaque it becomes.

Total WBC count:

$< 2,000$ mm³ · Non-inflammatory
May be seen in Systemic Lupus Erythematosus, systemic sclerosis, and crystalline arthropathy. Osteoarthrosis typically has a WBC count < 1000 mm³
$2,000 – 100,000$ mm³ - Intermediate range
Some joint sepsis can be in the 50K – 100K range, especially Gonococcal, TB, immune compromised host, partially treated infection. Likewise Crystalline arthropathies, rheumatoid arthritis, and Reiter's can also be in the 50 – 100K range.
$> 100,000$ mm³ · Septic joint until proven otherwise
The presence of crystals does not rule out infection with this presentation

Differential (% neutrophils)

< 50% - Non-inflammatory
< 90% - RA
> 95% - Infectious

> Gram Stain 50 - 75% sensitive
> (Do it yourself if necessary)
> Culture > 90% sensitive

Culture

Cultures are indispensable in directing antibiotic therapy. Sterile prep and handling are imperative!

---

34 Schmerling RH, et. al. Synovial Fluid Test: What should be ordered. JAMA 1990;264:1009-1014.

Polarized Microscopy

Monosodium Urate crystals (Gout) – Needle-shaped or long with blunt ends, strongly negative birefringent (brilliantly bright against a dark background)

Chondrocalcinosis crystals (CPPD) – Rod shaped/rhomboidal, weak positive birefringent.

Intra articular Betamethasone can mimic gout crystals.

Using polarized light microscopy
Gout - yellow when $\perp$, blue when $\parallel$ **CPPD** - opposite

Glucose (? significance)

Low glucose can be found in any joint with increased cellular activity within the joint. Thus it can be low in sepsis, RA, or crystalline arthropathies. To be useful it must also be compared to serum glucose. Glucose is limited in its ability to aid in the differentiation of infectious versus non-infectious etiologies.

String test (quantitative tests of viscosity don't support this test)

Inflammatory ($\downarrow$ viscosity) short string, Non-inflammatory ($\uparrow$ viscosity) long string

Tests for Infection

Gram Stain	
1. Heat fix slide until dry	4. Decolorizer 30 seconds
2. Gram violet x 1 minute, rinse	5. Safranin x 1 minute, rinse
3. Grams Iodine x 1 minute, rinse	6. Air dry

Tissue Frozen Section (Tissue biopsy the most inflammatory looking tissue)
0 Polymorphnuclear cells/high power field is evidence of the lack of infection
5 - 10 Polymorphnuclear cells/high power field is evidence of a probable infection[35]
> 10 Polymorphnuclear cells/high power field increases specificity to 99%[36]

Nerves, EMG, & NCV

EMG Findings/Meaning

Finding	Significance
Fibrillation potential at rest, Positive sharp waves	Partial denervation
Polyphasic motor units	Chronic denervation
New motor units	Nerve regeneration
No action potential	Complete lesion

EMG/NCV Normal values

	Distal latency (m sec.)	Amplitude(mv)
Median (motor/sensory)	2.4 - 4.4 / 2.5 - 3.7	4 - 18 / > 0.02
Ulnar (motor/sensory)	1.8 - 3.5 / 2.5 - 3.7	6 - 16 / > 0.02
Radial (sensory)	2.4 - 2.7	> 0.012

[35] Mirra JM, et al. The pathology of failed total joint Arthroplasty. Clin. Orthop. 1982;170:175-183.

[36] Lohner JH, et al. The reliability of analysis of intraoperative frozen sections for identifying active infection during revision hip or knee Arthroplasty. J Bone Joint Surg 1996;78A:1553-1558.

Electrodiagnostic Findings in Various Peripheral Nerve Disorders

	Root Lesion	Plexus Lesion	Focal Entrapment	Axonal Poly-neuropathy	De-myelinating Poly-neuropathy
Finding					
Motor Nerve Amplitude	+/- ↓	↓ (focal)	+/- ↓	↓(diffuse)	+/- ↓
Sensory Nerve Amplitude	Normal	↓ (focal)	+/- ↓	↓(diffuse)	+/- ↓
Distal Latency	Normal	Normal	↑ (focal)	Normal	↑(diffuse)
Conduction Velocity	Normal	Normal	↓ (focal)	Normal	↑(diffuse)
Fibrillations	+ (acute)	+ (acute)	+/- (severe)	+	+/-
Large Polyphasic MUAP's	+ (chronic)	+ (chronic)	+/- (severe)	+	+/-

Adapted from Robinson LR. Role of Neurophysiologic Evaluation in Diagnosis. J Am Acad Orthop Surg 2000;8:195

Nerve Injury Classification[37,38]

Seddon	Sunderland	Pathologic Findings
Neuropraxia	1	Localized myelin damage (Compression)
Axonotmesis	2	Loss of axonal continuity; endo-, peri-, and epineurium intact
	3	Axonal and endoneurial continuity lost
	4	Axonal, endoneurial, perineurial continuity lost
Neurotmesis	5	Complete nerve lesion

Wound Healing Indices (for normal healing)	Malnutrition
Serum Albumin > 3.5 g/dl	Total lymphocyte count < 1500/cubic mm
Absolute lymphocyte count > 1500/mm^3	Serum albumin < 3.5 gm/dL
Absolute doppler pressure 70 mmHg	Serum transferrin level < 226 mg/dL
Differential pressure index (ABI) > 0.5	
TcpO$_2$ 30 mm Hg	

[37] Sunderland S. Nerve injuries on their repair: A critical appraisal. NY: Churchill Livingstone, 1991.

[38] Seddon HJ. Surgical disorders of the peripheral nerves. Balt: Williams and Wilkins, 1972, pp 68-88.

Pediatric Medications

Analgesics (All doses mg/kg unless otherwise noted)

MEDICATION	PRODUCT	DOSAGE	ROUTE	MAXIMUM
acetaminophen Drops	80mg/0.8ml	10 - 15 Q4 - 6 hrs	PO	5 dose/day
acetaminophen Elixir	160mg/5ml		PO	5 dose/day
acetaminophen Chew	80 mg		PO	5 dose/day
acetaminophen Tabs	325mg		PO	5 dose/day
aspirin	81 mg	10 - 15 Q4 - 6 hrs	PO	
ibuprofen	100mg/5ml	5 - 10 q6 - 8h	PO	40 mg/kg/d
acetaminophen elixir/ codeine	120mg Acet/12mg Codeine/5ml	3 – 6 yo: 5 mL 7 - 12: 10 mL q4 - 6h		
diazepam		0.12 - .08 mg/kg/d divided TID - QID	PO/PR	
		0.04 - 0.2 q2 - 4hr	IV/IM	0.6 per 8 hr
demerol		1 - 1.8	IV/SC/PO slow IV	
morphine		0.1 - 0.2	IV/IM/SC	15 mg q4h
		0.1 - 0.2	PO	
codeine		0.5 - 1.2 Q4h	PO	$\geq$ 1 year

Antihistamines

hydroxizine	10 mg/5 ml	0.5 QID	PO	
diphenhydramine	12.5 mg/5mL 25,50 mg	5 mg/kg/d Divided QID	PO/IV/IM	300 mg/day

Helpful Pediatric Milestones and Angles

Gait	
Sitting - 6 months	Runs - 18 months
Cruises - 12 months (variable)	**Mature Gait - 3 - 5 years**
Independent walking - 15 months	

Rotational Profile

Foot progression angle: 5 - 20° external rotation	**Maximum varus** ~ Birth **Genu rectus** ~ 18 months **Maximum valgus** ~ 3 years
Hip Internal rotation: 30 - 60° (<20° femoral anteversion)	**Femoral Anteversion** 1 years – 31 degrees
Hip External rotation: 20 - 60° (>70° femoral anteversion)	8 years – 24 degrees 15 years - 15 degrees
Thigh foot angle: 0 - 20° external rotation (< negative 10° tibial torsion)	(Improves 15 degrees up to 15 years old)

Reflexes

Reflex	Disappears
Hand grasping	2 - 4 months
Plantar grasping	1 year
Moro	4 - 6 months
Stepping	1 - 2 months
Crossed extension	1 month
Withdrawal	Should always be present
Positive support response	4 months
Extensor thrust	2 months
Symmetrical tonic neck	present by 6 months, no absolute time for disappearance
Parachute	present by 6 months, persists through life

Characteristics of Myelodysplasia Levels

Level	Hip	Knee	Feet	Orthosis	Ambulation
L1	External rotation/ flexion	-	Equinovarus	HKAFO	Non
L2	Adduction/ flexion	Flexed	Equinovarus	HKAFO	Non
L3	Adduction/ flexion	Recurvatum	Equinovarus	KAFO	Household
L4	Adduction/ flexion	Extension	Cavovarus	AFO	Household +
L5	flexion	Limited flexion	Calcaneo-valgus	AFO	Community
S1				Shoes	Near normal

Adapted from Miller MD (ed.): <u>Review of Orthopaedics</u>, 3rd ed. Philadelphia, WB Saunders, 2000, page 160, with permission

Growth Plates

Upper Extremity (Range in parenthesis)

Growth Plate	Appearance	Closure
Medial clavicle	17	18 - 24
Acromion	15 - 18	18 - 19
Coracoid	1	18 - 21
Scapular body	1st fetal week	20 - 21
Glenoid	18	19
Humeral head	birth - 3 mo	Head and tuberosities 4 - 6 Fuse with shaft ♂:19 - 21, ♀:18 - 20
Greater tuberosity	♂:1/2 - 1, ♀:1/4 - 1.5	"
Lesser tuberosity	3 - 5	"
Lateral epicondyle	♂:12, ♀:11	Shaft, capitellum, trochlea 13 - 17 Fuse with shaft ♂:17, ♀:14
Capitellum	♂:5 mo., ♀:4 mo (6 wk - 8 mo)	"
Medial epicondyle	♂:5 - 7, ♀:3 - 6 (3-7)	♂:18, ♀:15
Olecranon	♂:10, ♀:8	♂:15 - 17, ♀:14 - 15
Radial head	♂:5, ♀:4 (3 - 6)	♂:15 - 17, ♀:14 - 15
Radial tuberosity	10 - 12	14 - 18
Distal radius	3 mo - 1.5 (3 mo - 1.5)	♂:19, ♀:17
Distal ulna	♂:6, ♀:5 (4 - 9)	♂:19, ♀:17
Scaphoid	♂:5.5, ♀:4.5 (2.5 - 9)	Variable
Lunate	4 (6 mo - 9.5)	Variable
Triquetrum	♂:2.25, ♀:1.75 (6 mo - 4)	Variable
Pisiform	♂:11, ♀:9	Variable
Trapezium	♂:5, ♀:4 (1.5 - 10)	Variable
Trapezoid	♂:6, ♀:4 (2.5 - 9)	Variable
Hamate	6 mo (0 - 1.5)	Variable
Capitate	6 mo (0 - 1)	Variable
Proximal thumb metacarpal	♂:2.5, ♀:1.66 (1 - 3.5)	14 - 21
Proximal thumb P1	5 mo - 2.5	14 - 21
Proximal thumb distal phalanx	♂:1.5, ♀:1	14 - 21
Distal I/M/R/S metacarpal	1 - 1.5	14 - 21
Proximal P1	5 mo - 2.5	14 - 21

Upper Extremity (Continued)

Growth Plate	Appearance	Closure
Proximal PII	5 mo - 2.5	14 - 21
Proximal PIII	5 mo - 2.5	14 - 21

Growth Plates Lower Extremity

	Appearance	Closure
Iliac crest	Puberty	fuse at puberty
Iliac tubercle Ischial spine	13 - 15	fuse at puberty
Pubic tubercle	18 - 20	fuse at puberty
Acetabulum	10 - 13	fuse at puberty
Ischial spine	13 - 15	fuse at puberty
Femoral Head	4 mo	♂:17 - 18, ♀:16 - 17
Greater trochanter	3	16 - 17
Lesser trochanter	♂:12, ♀:11	16 - 17
Distal Femur	36th fetal week	♂:18 - 19, ♀:17
Proximal tibia	40th fetal week	♂:18 - 19, ♀:16-17
Tibial tuberosity	7 - 15	19
Proximal fibula	♂:4, ♀:3	♂:18 - 20, ♀:16 - 18
Distal tibia	6 mo	17 - 18 (med. mal. 16 - 18)
Distal fibula	♂:1, ♀:9 mo	17 - 18
Calcaneus	24 - 26 fetal week	12 - 22
Talus	26 - 28 fetal week	Variable
Cuboid	40 fetal week	Variable
Navicular	♂:3, ♀:2	Variable
Cuneiforms	3 mo - 2	Variable
Metatarsal/Phalanges		18

Development of Cervical Spine

Age	Feature
< 6 mo	C1 body invisible and all synchondroses are open, vertebrate are normally wedged anteriorly, and there is often no lordosis to the non-injured spine
1 yr	Body of C1 becomes visible radiographically
3 yr	Posteriorly located spinous process synchondroses fuse Dens becomes ossified (visible radiographically)
3 - 6 yr	Neurocentral (body) and C2-odontoid synchondroses fuse Summit ossification center appears at the apex (top) of the odontoid Anterior wedging of the vertebral bodies resolve (and is not normal if seen)
8 yr	Pseudosubluxation and predental widening resolve, lordosis is normal now
12 - 14 yr	Secondary ossification centers appear at spinous process tips, summit ossification center of odontoid fuses (if it does not *os odontoideum* occurs), superior/inferior epiphyseal rings appear on dens
25 yr	Secondary ossification centers at tips of spinous processes fuse Superior/inferior epiphyseal rings fuse to vertebral body

Foot Deformities

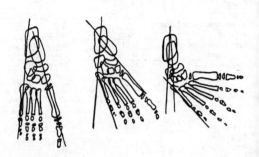

Normal   Metatarsus Adductus   Talipes Equinovarus

Angles and Characteristics

	Metatarsus Adductus	Talipes Equinovarus
Talo-calcaneal angle	20 - 40°	< 20°
Characteristics	adducted forefoot	talus and calcaneus **parallel**

Normal Talo-Calcaneal angle is 20 - 40°

	Calcaneovalgus	Metatarsus varus	Clubfoot
+ Dorsiflexion	Yes	Yes	No
Shape of sole	Deviates laterally	Deviates medially	Deviates medially
	"Banana"	"Kidney"	"Kidney"
Heel position	Valgus	Valgus	Varus

Brachial Plexus Birth Injuries

Name	Roots	Loss	Prognosis
Erb-Duchenne	C5/6	Deltoid, elbow flexors, dorsiflexion at hand/wrist, *"waiter's tip deformity"*	Best
Klumpke	C8/T1	Hand intrinsics, wrist flexors	Poor
Total Plexus	C5 -T1	Flaccid arm, sensory and motor loss	Worst

2:1000 births, Clavicle and proximal humerus fractures may mimic with pseudo-paralysis. Treat by maintaining Passive ROM. Return may be up to 18 months. NO biceps function at 3 months is an **ominous sign**.

Salter-Harris Classification of Physeal Injuries[39]

Type	Description	Characteristics
I	Transverse through growth plate	Younger age
II	Same as I with a metaphyseal fragment (Thurston-Holland fragment)	Older age (>10)
III	Through growth plate with extension through epiphysis into joint	Intra-articular
IV	Through epiphysis and metaphysis	Growth arrest
V	Crush injury to the growth plate	Late growth arrest
VI	Damage to the perichondral ring of LaCroix	Physeal bridge/ asymmetric growth irregularity (angular deformity)

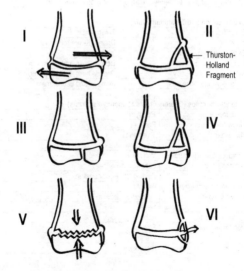

---

[39] Salter RB, Harris WR. Injuries involving the epiphyseal plate. J Bone Joint Surg 1963;45A:587-622

Night Pains (awakens child at night, gone during the daytime)

Localized pain (short Differential)	
Leukemia	Osteoid osteoma
Generalized pain (long Differential)	
Spinal dysraphism or tether	Knee – osteochondritis
Skeletal tumor	Feet – deformity
Fibrous dysplasia	Perthes disease of the hips
Muscle – hemangioma	Joints- arthritis
Subacute osteomyelitis	Kohler's disease

Osteochondritis Dessicans	
Knee and elbow most common (throwers)	trauma, ischemia,
(Lateral aspect of medial femoral condyle)	abnormal ossification
(Capitellum [Panner's disease])	10 -15 years
Activity related pain, tenderness, effusion	May be poly-articular

Classification and Treatment (Guhl)

Classification	Treatment
Intact	Drilling (K-wire retrograde)
Early-separated lesion	In-situ pinning
Partially detached lesion	Debride base, reduce, pinning
Salvageable loose body	Debride base, reduce, pinning
Unsalvageable loose body	Removal and debridement

Osteochondroses (Osteonecrosis at apophysis/physis)

Location	Eponym
Elbow (capitellum)	Panner's
Phalanges (hand)	Thiemann's
Spine	Scheuermann's
Ischiopubic synchondrosis	Van Neck's
Femoral head	Legg-Calve-Perthes
Inferior patella	Sinding-Larsen-Johansson
Proximal tibial epiphysis	Blount's
Tibial tuberosity	Osgood-Schlatter's
Calcaneus	Sever's
Tarsal navicular	Kohler's
Metatarsal head	Freiberg's
Scaphoid	Preiser's
Lunate	Kienbock's

Back Pain in Children: Diagnostic workup according to symptom severity

Level	Circumstance	Studies Recommended
I	Minor trauma No systemic signs (fever) Negative physical exam	Often none Follow up 1-2 weeks
II	History unclear No systemic signs (fever) Minor exam findings (tight hamstrings, spinal asymmetry)	Radiographs AP/lateral lumbosacral obliques
III	History unclear May have systemic signs (fever) Often significant exam findings (tight hamstrings, +SLR, spinal asymmetry)	Radiographs AP/lateral CBC, ESR bone scan (if ESR elevated)
IV	History Unclear, Often have systemic signs (fever), marked exam findings, to include neurological deficit	Radiographs AP/lateral CBC, ESR, bone scan MRI, CT, or both

Adapted with permission from Wenger DR, Mercer R: The Art and Practice of Children's Orthopaedics. Lippincott-Williams & Wilkins, 1993, page 457

Mucopolysaccharidosis

Syndrome	Inheritance	Intelligence	Cornea	Urinary Excretion
I. Hurler's (Worst)	Autosomal recessive	Mental retardation	Cloudy	Dermatan/Heparan Sulphate
II. Hunter's	X-linked recessive	Mental retardation	Clear	Dermatan/Heparan Sulphate
III. Sanfilippo's	Autosomal recessive	Mental retardation	Clear	Heparan Sulphate
IV. Morquio's (Commonest)	Autosomal recessive	Normal	Cloudy	Keratan Sulphate

Scheuermann's Kyphosis[40] (Thoracic)

Kyphosis > 45°, 5° or more anterior wedging at 3 consecutive vertebrae
  Other radiographic findings = disc narrowing, end-plate changes, spondylolysis
  (30 - 50%), scoliosis (33%), and Schmorl's nodes
♂ more common, Adolescents with poor posture and occasionally aching pain
Hyperkyphosis that does not improve with hyperextension (if hyperkyphosis
  improves with hyperextension diagnosis = postural kyphosis, tight hamstrings
Brace progressive curves (Risser 1 - 3), > 1 year, may improve curve
Risser 5, >75°, consider fusion

Lumbar Scheuermann's – Athletes/manual laborers, less common, end plate changes, Schmorl's nodes, ↓ disc height, lacks wedging, mechanical back pain.
Usually Self Limited

---

[40] Lowe TG. Current Concepts Review: Scheuermann's disease. J Bone Joint Surg 1990;72A:940-945.

Dysplasia	Inheritance	Zone	Clinical Findings	Radiologic Features
Achondroplasia	AD/SM	Epiphyseal	Abnormal facies and spine	Lumbar stenosis bow legs
Pseudoachondroplasia	AD	Epiphyseal	Normal facies, atlantoaxial instability, scoliosis, early OA	Metaphyseal flaring, delayed epiphyseal ossification, hypoplastic dens
SED (Congenita)	AD/SM	Epiphyseal	Flattened facies	Platyspondyly, delayed epiphysis
SED (tarda)	XR	Epiphyseal	Kyphosis, hip pain	Platyspondyly, dysplastic dens
Chondrodysplasia punctata	AD (fatal)	Physeal	Flat facies	Stippled epiphysis
Kniest Syndrome	AD	Physeal	Detached retina, scoliosis, cleft palate	Dumbbell femurs, osteopenia/hypoplasia
Metaphyseal chondrodysplasia	AD/AR	Metaphyseal	Wide eyes, bow legs	Bowed legs
Multiple epiphyseal dysplasia	AD	Epiphyseal	Delayed ambulation – waddling gait	Irregular epiphyseal ossification
Dysplasia epiphysealis hemimelica (Trevor's)	–	Metaphyseal	Bow legs	Hemi-enlarged epiphysis
Progressive diaphyseal dysplasia	AD	Diaphyseal	Delayed walking	Symmetrical cortical thickening
Mucopolysaccharidosis	AR/XR	Hypophyseal	Corneal changes, urinary sugars, cauliflower ears, hitchhiker thumb, rigid clubfoot	Thick bone, bullet shaped metacarpals
Diastrophic dysplasia	AR	Physeal	Cleft palate, cauliflower ears, hitchhiker thumb, rigid clubfoot	Kyphoscoliosis, odontoid hypoplasia
Cleidocranial dysplasia	AD	Metaphyseal	Absent clavicles, wide cranial sutures	Delayed physeal closure

AD Autosomal dominant, SM Spontaneous mutation, AR Autosomal Recessive,
XR X-linked recessive, SED Spondyloepiphyseal dysplasia, OA Osteoarthrosis

Modified from Miller MD (ed.) Review of Orthopaedics. 3rd ed. Philadelphia, WB. Saunders, 2000, p.151 with permission

Disproportionate

Proportionate

Slipped Capital Femoral Epiphysis[41]

-Prevalence 0.2 / 100,000 (Japan) to 10.08 / 100,000 (Northeastern US)	
-60% male	-50% > 95th percentile for weight
-Mean age = 13.5 in boys 12 in girls	-Bilaterality as high as 63%

Classification

Pre-slip	Acute (10-15%)	Chronic (85%)	Acute-on-chronic

Stable - walk without crutches (nearly 0% avascular necrosis)
Unstable - can't walk without crutches (up to 50% avascular necrosis)

Radiographs

Show a superior and anterior slip of the proximal femoral metaphysis with respect to the capital femoral epiphysis. In a gradual slip you may see superior and anterior remodeling on the femoral metaphysis and periosteal new bone formation.

Physical Exam

Flexed and externally rotated position, may mimic fracture in pain/presentation
(May be considered a Salter Harris I of the proximal femoral physis)

Metaphyseal Blanch sign of Steel AND Klein's line

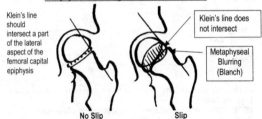

Klein's line should intersect a part of the lateral aspect of the femoral capital epiphysis

Klein's line does not intersect

Metaphyseal Blurring (Blanch)

No Slip   Slip

Ultrasound can be used to look for effusion and periosteal bone formation (unstable)
MRI and bone scans may also be utilized

Grading

Slips <30° mild, 30-50° moderate, >50° severe
Good results with in-situ pinning with mild and moderate slips

Treatment

In situ pinning favored – single pin under fluoroscopic guidance (still controversial especially with respect to traction, reduction)
Treatments ranging from hip spica casting to osteotomies have been proposed

---

[41] Loder RT, et al. Slipped Capital Femoral Epiphysis. JBJS 2000;82A:1185.

Ranges of values for the differential diagnoses of the child with a limp

Condition	Complete Blood Count	Erythrocyte Sedimentation Rate Following trend useful	Tc99 Bone scan Increased vascularity = Increased uptake
Transient synovitis	↔ , mild ↑	↔ , mild ↑	↑
Slipped Capital Femoral Epiphysis	↔ , mild ↑	↔ , mild ↑	
Herniated Nucleus Polposus	↔ , mild ↑	↔ , mild ↑	
Spondylolithesis, spondylolysis	↔ , mild ↑	↔ , mild ↑	
Pauciarticular Juvenile Rheumatoid Arthritis (JRA)	↔ , mild ↑		
Lyme disease	↔ , mild ↑	↑	
Pyarthrosis	↑	↑	↑
Osteomyelitis	↑	↔ , mild ↑	↑
Soft tissue abscess/Cellulitis	↑	↑	↔ , mild ↑
Acute rheumatic fever	↑	↑	
Polyarticular/systemic JRA	↑	↑	↑
Discitis	↑	↑	↑
Trauma	↔	↔ , mild ↑	↑ (Subacute) ↑ (Stress fracture)

NOTE: Look for left shift with pyogenic process, platelets may elevate as an acute phase reactant.
NOTE: Fluid collection in joint may obscure uptake giving a false negative.
Gallium localizes WBC collections better

Radiographs
    Obtain spine, pelvis, and extremity
    Periosteal reaction ~ 2 weeks
    Medial joint space increased > 2 mm in hip is significant.
    Endosteal erosion, disc space mineralization in discitis

Ultrasound
    Less invasive, easy to get, operator dependent

MRI
    Good for soft tissue and differential between dead and living bone.
    Early Perthes, evaluate spinal cord and disc

Limp – Differential Diagnosis

Toddlers	4 - 10 years	11 - 16 years
Developmental hip dysplasia	Perthes	Slipped capital femoral epiphysis
Mild cerebral palsy	Osteomyelitis	Toxic synovitis
Toddlers fracture	Septic hip/joint	DDH (untreated)
Juvenile RA	Leg length difference > 1 - 2 inch	Tumor
Discitis		Tarsal coalition
		Toxic synovitis

A hip radiograph is invaluable for any child with a limp and without an obvious etiology

---

Osteomyelitis in Children

See antibiotic section for choice of antibiotics and common pathogens.
Usually via a blood-borne route. Rarely crosses the physis (subacute osteomyelitis can) and usually resides in the metaphysis or epiphysis due to vascular anatomy.
Physical exam may show pain, loss of function, erythema, warmth, and occasionally abscess.

Discitis

Refusal to walk or sit, Decreased ROM of spine, MRI is diagnostic early
Radiographs may show late disc space narrowing
Treat: Bed rest (no traction), immobilization, +/- antibiotics

Genu Varum

Disorder of the posterior medial physis
Blount's disease = Drennan's angle > 11°
Metaphyseal beaking
African-American, Obese Common

Metaphyseal-diaphyseal angle

Treatment Based on Age and Langinskiold's Stages

Age	Stage	Treatment
<18 month	I - II	None
18 - 24 months	I - II	Night bracing
2 - 3 years	I - II	Daytime brace
3 - 8 years	III - V	Osteotomy
3 - 8 years	VI (bony bridge)	Resection of bony bridge

> Remember: Knee pain could be hip pathology
> Limp can be spine pathology
> Refusal to walk or sit may be either

Scoliosis
Neuromuscular Scoliosis
Common in neuromuscular conditions, may progress rapidly, may progress after
maturation, often associated with pelvic obliquity, bony deformities, and
involvement of the cervical spine

Infantile Idiopathic Scoliosis

2 months - 3 years	Other associated defects
Left sided thoracic	Most common in United Kingdom
Male predominance	Curve < 20°, rib vertebral angle difference < 20° resolve
Skull flattening	MRI severe curves

Juvenile Idiopathic Scoliosis

- 3 - 10 years	- 70% need treatment
- High risk for progression	- 50% surgery
	- 50% bracing

Adolescent Idiopathic Scoliosis
Progression v. Magnitude/Skeletal Maturity (Lonstein/Carlson)[42]
(expressed in percentage of progression)

Risser Sign	5-19 Degree	20-29 Degree
1-2	22%	68%
2-4	1.6%	23%

> Scoliometer threshold = 7°, Progression = Increased Cobb angle >5°
> (Curve apex < T8 use Boston bucket, > T7 use Boston + Milwaukee)
> Hard or difficult to brace hypokyphosis/thoracic lordosis in a brace

Treatment Guidelines

Curve	Progression	Risser stage	Therapy
0 – 25°	-	0 - 4	Serial observation
25 - 30°	5 - 10°	0 - 4	Brace (halt or slow progression)
30 - 40°	-	0 - 4	Brace (halt or slow progression)
> 40°	-	0 - 4	Surgery *
> 50°	-	5	Surgery (young adults)

*Posterior spinal fusion, Add anterior spinal fusion for > 75°, ♀ <10, ♂ < 13

---

42 Lonstein JE and Carlson JM. The prediction of curve progression in untreated idiopathic scoliosis during growth. JBJS 66:1067, 1984

Progression risk factors (Curve > 20°, < 12 years, Risser 0 - 1 at presentation)

MR imaging criteria/Rapid Progression (Tumor, tethered cord, Syringomyelia)	
- Structural abnormality in plain films	- Pain
- Excessive Kyphosis	- Left thoracic curve & focal neuro finding
- Juvenile onset (< 11)	- Radiographic abnormality
- Abnormal neurologic exam	- Associated syndromes

King Curves (Patterns of Idiopathic Scoliosis)[43]

Type	Definition	Flexibility
I	S-shaped thoracolumbar curve, crosses midline	Lumbar > thoracic
II	S-shaped thoracolumbar curve, crosses midline	Lumbar < thoracic
III	Right thoracic curve, T4 does not tilt into the curve	Lumbar vertebrae highly flexible
IV	Long thoracic curve, T4 tilts into the curve	L4 tilts to thoracic curve
V	Double thoracic curve	T1 tilts to upper curve

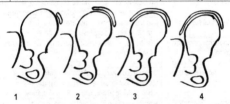

   1   2   3   4

Risser Stages (5 = fusion of iliac apophysis)

Congenital Spinal Deformities

Associated with genitourinary abnormalities (25%), cardiac (10%), and dysraphism (25% - commonly diastomatomyelia)

Risk of Progression	Curve progression
Unilateral unsegmented bar & contralateral hemivertebrae	Rapid & relentless
Unilateral unsegmented bar	Rapid
Fully segmented hemivertebrae	Steady
Partially segmented hemi vertebrae	Less rapid, < 40° at maturity
Incarcerated hemivertebrae	None or slow
Non-segmented hemivertebrae	Little

Top 3 usually need surgery, Bottom three can be observed – partially segmented hemivertebrae will sometimes need excision

---

[43] King HA, Moe JH, Bradford DS, et al. The selection of fusion levels in thoracic idiopathic scoliosis. J Bone Joint Surg 1983;83-A:1302-1313.

Skeletal Survey in Child abuse

AP bilateral hands, forearms, arms, thighs, legs, and feet
AP/lateral axial skeleton and trunk
AP/lateral skull

Differential Diagnosis in Child Abuse

Diagnosis	Factors and/or characteristics
Accident	Age, mechanism of injury, assoc. injuries, no delay in seeking care
Birth trauma	Obstetric history, callus within 2 weeks of birth, humeral or clavicle fracture, distal humeral physeal separation
Osteogeneis imperfecta	Family history, osteopenia, blue sclera, dental abnormalities, wormian bones, skin-test abnormalities
Caffey's disease	Family history, Diffuse periosteal elevation, mandibular involvement, irritability, inflammation, swelling, stiffness
Rickets	Physeal widening, metabolic abnormalities, deformity, osteopenia, Looser's lines, laboratory abnormalities
Congenital syphilis	Metaphyseal erosions, periosteal bone formation, positive serological tests, pseudoparalysis
Congenital insensitivity to pain "Riley-Day syndrome"	Infection, joint destruction, neurologic abnormalities, family history
Coagulation disorders	Bruising, coagulopathy, laboratory abnormalities
Leukemia	Metaphyseal lucencies, systemic symptoms, hematologic abnormalities, + bone marrow biopsy
Normal radiographic variants	Angulation of ossifying metaphysis, cortical irregularities, spurring, juxtaphyseal variants

Adapted from Kocher MS, Kasser JR: Orthopedic Aspects of Child Abuse. J Am Acad Orthop Surg 2000;8:10-20

Specificity of Musculoskeletal Findings in Child Abuse

High specificity	Metaphyseal corner lesions, posterior rib, scapular, spinous process, or sternal fractures
Moderate specificity	Multiple fractures, fractures of different ages, epiphyseal separations, vertebral body, digital, or complex skull fractures
Low specificity (but common in child abuse)	Clavicular, long-bone shaft, or linear skull fractures

Legg-Calves-Perthes Disease
Osteonecrosis of the proximal femoral epiphysis
Boys 4 - 8, Delayed skeletal maturation

Legg - Calves - Perthes Stages

Stage	Characteristics
Initial	Physeal irregularity, metaphyseal blurring, radiolucencies
Fragmentation	Radiolucencies and radiodensities
Reossification	Normal density returns
Healed	Residual deformity

Classification schemes

Caterall	Salter & Thompson	Location (lateral view)	Prognosis
I	A	Anterior	Good
II	A	Anterior and partial lateral	Good
III	B	Anterior and lateral margin	Poor
IV	B	Epiphyseal dome - all	Poor

(based on amount of femoral involvement)

> **Risks** - positive family history, low birth weight, abnormal birth presentation
> **Physical signs** - Trendelenburg gait, hip or knee pain, decreased range of motion (especially abduction and Internal rotation)
> **Key to prognosis** - age > 6 years = worse
> **Bilateral 12 - 15%**

Herrings Lateral Pillar Classification (Group) and Goals/Recommendations[44]

Age	Group	Goals	Recommendations (HIGHLY controversial)
< 6	Any	Symptomatic relief	NSAID's, home traction, limit weight bearing
6 - 8	A	Symptomatic relief	Same as above
	B	Containment	Traction, muscle releases, abduction brace, osteotomies
	C	Containment	Same as B, bracing ineffective due to difficulty centering capital femoral epiphysis
≤ 9	A	Symptomatic relief	NSAID's, home traction, limit weight bearing
	B	Containment	Bracing difficult due to loss of motion and poor compliance
	C	Containment	Osteotomies, muscle releases, Petrie cast

Herring Classification:[45] A – normal pillar height, B - > 50% height, C - < 50%

[44] Herring JA. Current Concepts Review: The treatment of Legg-Calves-Perthes Disease. JBJS 76A:448-457,1994.
[45] Herring JA, et al. The lateral pillar classification of Legg-Calves-Perthes disease JPO 12:143-150, 1992.

Developmental Dysplasia of the Hip (DDH) (Risk = 1:1000)
Associated conditions - Metatarsus adductus, clubfoot, calcaneovalgus, torticollis
Increased in Native Americans and Laplanders
Rare in African descent

Risk with history:	
6%	normal parents 1 affected kid
12%	1 affected parent no kids
36%	1 affected parent 1 kid

80% female
Left 60%, Right 20%, Both 20%
Increased with breech firstborn;
2x as common as subsequent sibs

Radiographs may be confirmatory, but not definitely excluded
If subluxation suspected dynamic ultrasound may be helpful

Algorithm for evaluation and treatment of DDH[46]

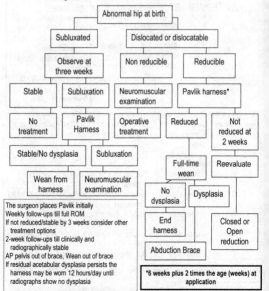

The surgeon places Pavlik initially
Weekly follow-ups till full ROM
If not reduced/stable by 3 weeks consider other treatment options
2-week follow-ups till clinically and radiographically stable
AP pelvis out of brace, Wean out of brace
If residual acetabular dysplasia persists the harness may be worn 12 hours/day until radiographs show no dysplasia

*6 weeks plus 2 times the age (weeks) at application

[46] Guille JT, Pizzutillo MD, and MacEwen GD. Developmental Dysplasia of the Hip from Birth to Six Months. JAAOS 1999;8:232-242.

Physical Exam

Hand

Test	Description	Positive Findings
Carpal tunnel compression	Direct pressure over the carpal tunnel just distal to distal wrist flexion crease, 30 – 60 sec.	Reproduces median nerve symptoms
Tinel's	Tap directly over peripheral nerve, symptoms in distribution of nerve	Nerve irritation, neuroma
Phalen's	Volar flex wrist ~ 30 - 60s, Reproduces median nerve findings	Median nerve compression
Elbow flexion	Hyper flexion elbow ~ 30 - 60 seconds, reproduces ulnar nerve symptoms	Ulnar nerve compression
Finkelstein's	Make fist, thumb in palm, ulnar flex wrist. Reproduces pain in 1st dorsal compartment	DeQuervain's tenosynovitis
Allen's	Compress radial and ulnar arteries at wrist, make fist, relax fist, release arteries one at a time, shows ulnar and radial artery patency (Can be performed on fingers)	Arterial patency in the hand
Spurling's	Axial load skull with the neck in extension and deviation to the symptomatic side – worsens nerve root compression	Nerve root compression, radicular pain
Flexor digitorum profundus	Hyper extend MCPJ, lock PIPJ in extension, have patient flex DIPJ	Tendon continuity
Flexor digitorum superficialis	Isolate finger by extending all others, have patient flex finger. Flex finger with metacarpophalangeal joint extended otherwise hand intrinsics contribute.	Tendon continuity
Tenodesis effect	Flex wrist – fingers extend. Extend wrist – fingers flex (resting tone – intact tendons)	Tendon continuity
Passive test of continuity	Flex wrist, grasp forearm just proximal to wrist flexion crease, squeezing here will flex fingers	Tendon continuity
Froment's	Have patient pinch a piece of paper, Weak pinch & flexion of DIPJ of thumb signifies ulnar neuropathy (weak adductor pollicis and flexor pollicis brevis)	Ulnar neuropathy
Watson test	Thumb over volar distal pole of scaphoid, radial deviation of wrist flexes scaphoid, with torn scapholunate ligament the lunate moves volar 'clunk' past scaphoid	Scapholunate Interosseus ligament tear
Regan test	Shucking ulnar wrist while stabilizing the lunate	Lunotriquetral ligament

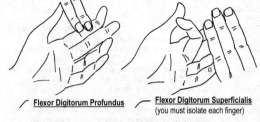

<u>Flexor Digitorum Profundus</u>   <u>Flexor Digitorum Superficialis</u>
                                          (you must isolate each finger)

| Quick Neurologic Assessment of the Hand |

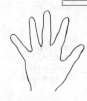

<u>Ulnar Nerve</u> –
Active finger abduction

<u>Anterior interosseous n.</u>
– flexor digitorum
profundus (index) & flexor
pollicis longus

<u>Posterior interosseous n.</u>
– extensor indicis proprius
and extensor digiti quinti
minimi

<u>Finger Block – Flexor tendon sheath block</u>

Direct volar injection midline and down to bone
over the A2 pulley. Slowly withdraw while
injecting. Inject when you feel a loss of
resistance to avoid injecting the substance of the
tendons. You can feel the fluid go into the flexor
sheath.

Digital nerve block may also be performed
by blocking the volar and dorsal sensory
branches at the level of the metacarpo-
phalangeal joint

Flexor Tendon Zones

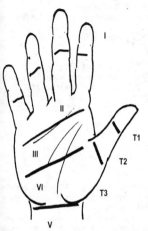

Flexor Zones
I. Distal to flexor digitorum superficialis insertion
II. Within finger flexor retinaculum ("No man's zone")
III. The palm
IV. Carpal Tunnel
V. Wrist and Forearm
T1. Distal to flexor pollicus longus insertion
T2. Thumb flexor retinaculum
T3. Thenar eminence

Extensor Zones
I. Distal Interphalangeal joint
II. Middle phalanx (PII)
II. Proximal Interphalangeal joint
III. Proximal phalanx (PI)
IV. Metacarpal phalangeal joint
V. Metacarpal
VI. Dorsal wrist
VII. Distal forearm
VIII. Mid/proximal forearm

Flexor sheaths, radial and ulnar bursa

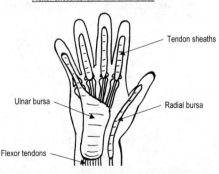

Tendon sheaths

Ulnar bursa

Radial bursa

Flexor tendons

Mallet Finger and Swan Neck Deformity

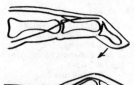

Mallet Finger-
Loss of continuity of terminal tendon
of extensor apparatus
Lacks ability to extend distal phalanx

Swan neck deformity-
Lax or disrupted volar plate, sagittal
band subluxate dorsal, distal
phalanx flexes, Proximal Interphalangeal joint hyper extends

Wrist Injection
- Inject dorsally through the fourth dorsal compartment aiming for the capito-lunate interval. Palpate/visualize the fluid entering the wrist joint.

Wrist Block
- Ulnar nerve- Inject radial to the flexor carpi ulnaris (FCU) at the proximal wrist flexion crease. Beware the ulnar artery just radial to the nerve. Raise a wheal ulnar to the FCU tendon to get the dorsal branch.
- Median nerve- Inject ulnar to the palmaris longus tendon at the distal wrist flexion crease. Angle needle 30 degrees to the skin aiming distally. Stop needle or injection for any median nerve symptoms.
- Radial nerve- Inject radial to the radial artery at the level of the radial styloid. Raise a wheal around dorsally and radially to get all the branches at this level.

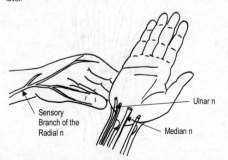

Sensory
Branch of the
Radial n

Ulnar n

Median n

Elbow

Test	Description	Positive Findings
Lateral pivot shift	Patient supine, elbow flexed, hold wrist in supination and apply valgus load, other hand hold forearm and adds an axial load	Apprehension = lateral collateral ligament insufficiency
Valgus instability	Valgus load applied to the extended elbow with the wrist in supination	Medial collateral ligament insufficiency
Tennis elbow	Pain just distal to the lateral epicondyle with resisted wrist extension	Lateral epicondylitis

Elbow Joint Injection/Aspiration

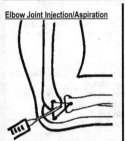

Inject in the center of the triangle formed by the radial head, lateral epicondyle, and the olecranon.

Carrying angle-
The angle formed by the arm and the forearm. Important to observe when treating elbow fractures in adults

Normally a variable valgus angulation

Lateral Pivot Shift test

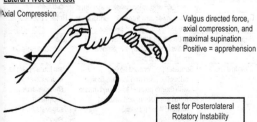

Axial Compression

Valgus directed force, axial compression, and maximal supination
Positive = apprehension

Test for Posterolateral Rotatory Instability

Shoulder

Test	Description	Positive Findings
Impingement	Passive forward flexion > 90 degrees	Pain = impingement
Hawkins	Impingement with internal rotation at 90° forward flexion	Pain = impingement
Impingement sign	No pain with test after subacromial injection	
Apprehension	90 degrees of abduction and external rotation, Apprehension of dislocation	Anterior capsular instability
Relocation	Supine apprehension, apprehension resolves with a posterior directed force on humerus	Anterior capsular instability
Load shift	Axially applied force to humerus while bringing the arm from straight lateral abduction to 90 degrees of forward flexion. Causes apprehension or posterior shift	Posterior capsular instability
Sulcus sign	Downward axial load to humerus subluxates humeral head inferiorly	Ligamentous laxity
Cross arm	Bring arm from 90 degrees forward flexion to across the chest, causing pain at acromioclavicular joint	Acromioclavicular arthrosis
Yergason's	Resisted supination, elbow at 90 degrees	Pain = bicipital tendonitis
Speed's	Yergason's with forward elevation	Pain = bicipital tendonitis
Lift-off sign	Patient lifts flat hand off back, ability to lift-off = intact subscapularis	Intact subscapularis
Horn blower's	Lifts arm up to 90° external rotation and 90° abduction, weak = abnormal	Posterior rotator cuff tear
Drop arm	Slowly lower arm from 90° abduction to the side, Drop arm is positive	Rotator cuff tear
Napoleon's	Hands flat on stomach, have patient actively keep elbows anterior to frontal plane of body	Intact subscapularis
O'Brien's	Shoulder 90° forward flexion, 30° adduction, resisted forward flexion with thumb pointed to ground, rotate to full supination, and resisted forward flexion again	Pain thumb pointed to ground and shoulder click with supination suggests SLAP* lesion

*SLAP = Superior labrum anterior posterior

Acromioclavicular joint injection

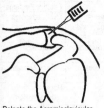

Palpate the Acromioclavicular joint, inject at 45 degrees to skin lateral to medial, joint should accept 1 - 1.5 cc of injection.

Subacromial Injection

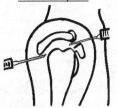

Palpate the Acromial arch. Inject under the arch from anterior or posterior.

Glenohumeral Joint Injection/Aspiration

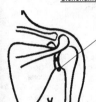

Injection point

Palpate the glenohumeral joint line from posterior about 2 cm inferior and 1 cm medial to the postero lateral acromion. Aim the needle towards the coracoid anteriorly.

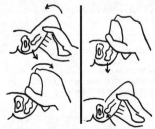

Barlow (Left) and Ortolani (Right) Tests

Hold thigh gently (like holding a tomato), don't press too hard on the thigh

Relaxation (the baby) is imperative, sleeping is perfect

Ortolani (out to in, O – I), Barlow the opposite!

Spine

Test	Description	Positive Findings
Hoffman's	Flicking DIPJ of middle finger causes involuntary flexion of DIPJ of index and IPJ of thumb	Myelopathic sign
Lhermitte's	Forward flexion of neck causes lancinating pain down spinal cord	Stenotic sign
Babinski	Stroking the bottom of the foot causes reflex toe extension	Upper motor neuron lesion
Clonus	Forced dorsiflexion of the foot	Reflex rhythmic plantar flexion response > 4 beats
Non-organic[47] signs *Waddell's signs*	1. Pain (out of proportion) to superficial touch [superficial tenderness] 2. Pain with axial rotation of the pelvis and with axial loading on the top of the skull [simulation] 3. Sitting straight leg raise < lying SLR [distraction] 4. Non anatomic weakness or sensory changes 5. Overreaction	May indicate heavy psychosocial overlay
Straight leg raise	Passive lifting of straight leg, flex hip with straight knee, ± dorsiflexion of foot (Lesegue maneuver)	Reproduces radicular symptoms, dorsiflexion should reproduce symptoms at less hip flexion
Crossed straight leg raise	Passive lifting of contralateral straight leg, flex hip with straight knee	98% specific for HNP
Bowstring	Hip flexed to 90°, knee flexed to reduce radicular symptoms, pressure placed on tibial nerve in popliteal area	Reproduces radicular pain
Femoral nerve traction test	Place the patient laterally on the unaffected side, examiner passively extends the hip and flexes the knee of the affected side	Reproduces radicular pain

---

[47] Wadell G, McCulloch JA, Kummel E, et al. Non organic physical signs in low back pain. Spine 5:117-125, 1980.

Hip

Test	Description	Positive Findings
Resisted straight leg raise	Active straight leg raise reproduces groin or low posterior buttock pain (also referred to as the Stinchfield test)	Hip irritability or arthrosis
FABER	Flexion, abduction, and external rotation may cause pain in sacroiliac joint, hip joint, or iliopsoas insertion	Sacroiliac joint, hip joint, tendonitis
Ortolani	Infant relaxed hips flexed, gently abduct, hip should relocate	Developmental hip dysplasia (DDH)
Barlow	Infant relaxed hips flexed, gently adduct, hip may sublux or dislocate	Subluxable or dislocatable DDH
Galeazzi	Infant relaxed and supine, feet flat, knees flexed. Asymmetric knee height = DDH	DDH, dislocated hip

Knee

Test	Description	Positive Findings
Varus/valgus at 30°	Flex knee 30° off exam table edge, stress varus and valgus	Valgus laxity = MCL Varus laxity = LCL
Same at 0°	Same at 0°	MCL/LCL & PCL or ACL
Lachman's	Pull tibia forward with respect to femur with knee flexed to 30°	Laxity = ACL injury Test symmetry
Anterior drawer	Pull tibia forward with knee at 90°	Same as above
Pivot shift	Take extended and internally rotated knee and flex with a valgus force, relocation = ACL injury	ACL injury Test symmetry
Posterior drawer	Knee flexed at 90 degrees, foot flat and fixed, posterior force on tibia. Subluxation of condyles towards or anterior to the anterior tibial margin = PCL laxity/deficiency	PCL injury or insufficiency
External rotation recurvatum	Pick up leg by great toes, knee goes into varus and recurvatum	Posterior lateral and PCL injury
Asymmetric external rotation	Patient prone, knees flexed at 90 degrees, externally rotate both feet at 30 and 90 degrees. Asymmetric external rotation > 10 - 15 degrees = posterolateral corner injury, if asymmetric at both 30 and 90 then PLC & PCL	PLC or PLC/PCL injury
Patellar apprehension	Laterally push patella with the knee in 20 - 30° of flexion	Apprehension = patellar dislocation or subluxation

Knee Injection

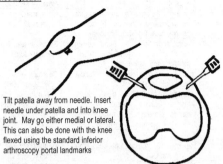

Tilt patella away from needle. Insert needle under patella and into knee joint. May go either medial or lateral. This can also be done with the knee flexed using the standard inferior arthroscopy portal landmarks

Ankle/Foot

Test	Description	Positive Findings
Ant. drawer	Knee flexed, quad relaxed, cup heel, stabilize tibia, pull forward on heel. Asymmetric anterior excursion = ankle instability	Asymmetric excursion = ankle instability
Talar tilt	Inversion at ankle causes tilting and lifting of the talus from the mortise.	Asymmetric excursion = ankle instability
Thompson's	Patient prone, knee flexed, squeezing calf should cause ankle plantar flexion	Absence of plantar flexion = achilles rupture
Ankle Squeeze test	Squeeze calf above syndesmosis, pain at syndesmosis or below = injury	High ankle sprain, syndesmosis injury
Coleman Block Test	Place a block under the lateral hindfoot, supple hindfoot deformities accommodate for the block, fixed do not	Fixed hindfoot deformity

Ankle Joint Injection

Palpate the joint line, direct needle at medial or lateral corner and under tibial plafond. Avoid saphenous vein medially, superficial peroneal nerve laterally, and the dorsalis pedis in the middle.

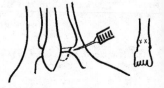

Hematoma Block

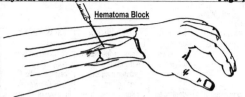

Palpate the fracture site. Inject indirectly onto the bone moving towards the fracture site until the anesthetic flows freely. Alternately inject and aspirate at the site (Barbotage). Used commonly for distal radius fractures.

Ankle Block

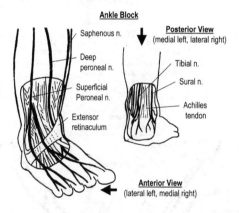

Saphenous n.

Deep peroneal n.

Superficial Peroneal n.

Extensor retinaculum

Posterior View
(medial left, lateral right)

Tibial n.

Sural n.

Achilles tendon

Anterior View
(lateral left, medial right)

- **Tibial nerve block** – inject behind the medial malleolus, halfway between the malleolus and the calcaneus.
- **Deep Peroneal nerve block** – inject lateral to the extensor hallucis longus and anterior tibial artery level with the inferior extensor retinaculum
- **Superficial Peroneal nerve block** – inject subcutaneously anterior to the extensor tendons
- **Saphenous nerve** – inject subcutaneously anterior to the medial malleolus
- **Sural nerve** – inject midway between the posterior border of the lateral malleolus and the calcaneus.

Radiologic Views
Spine

LINE / ANGLE	NORMAL	DESCRIPTION	SIGNIFICANCE
McCrae's Line	Odontoid tip should be below this line	Lateral C-spine: Diameter line drawn in the plane of the foramen magnum opening	Any existing compression will likely be asymptomatic if the tip is below this line
Chamberlain's Line	Odontoid tip <3mm above this line	Straight line from the posterior edge of the foramen magnum to the upper corner of the most posterior aspect of the hard palate	Intrusion of odontoid into foramen magnum
McGregor's Line	Odontoid tip not > 4.5 mm above this line	Upper corner of the most posterior aspect of the hard palate to the lowest border of the occipital skull.	Landmarks identifiable in all age groups

ADI = Atlanto dens interval
SAC = Space available for the cord

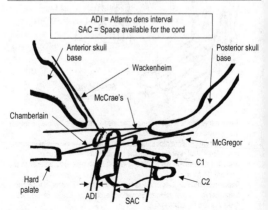

Spine

LINE / ANGLE	NORMAL	DESCRIPTION	SIGNIFICANCE
Space Avail. for Cord (SAC)	13 - 14mm at craniocervical junction; 12 mm below C2	Distance from posterior aspect of odontoid (craniocervical junction) or vertebral body (below C2) to the nearest posterior structure	Smaller distances indicative of cord compression
Pavlov's Ratio	> 0.8	Distance from the posterior margin of the vertebral body to the anterior margin of the spinous process divided by the distance from the anterior to the posterior margin of the vertebral body	< 0.8 is consistent with cervical stenosis
Atlanto Dens Interval (ADI) ADI increased with atlantoaxial instability (Down's Morquio's, Larsen's, Achondroplasia, SED)	3mm in adults 4mm in kids	Distance from the anterior odontoid to posterior border of the anterior arch of C1.	In trauma: 3-5mm: rupture of transverse ligament 5-10mm: alar ligament stretched 10-12mm: rupture of all ligaments
Power's Ratio	< 0.9 Normal	Ratio of lines drawn from Basion to C1 posterior arch and Opisthion to C1 anterior arch	> 1 Anterior atlanto-occipital dissociation
Scotty Dog	No collar	Oblique view of the Lumbar spine	Defect in the pars interarticularis
Sacral Inclination	Normal < 30°	Angle formed by a line drawn parallel to the posterior sacrum at S1 and one perpendicular to the floor	Risk for progression of slip
Slip Angle	< 10 °	Angle formed by a line perpendicular to the sacrum at S1 and the inferior endplate of L5	Risk for progression of slip if > 10°
Cobb Angle	0°	Cobb method is the method chosen by the Scoliosis Research Society for measuring and following scoliotic curves. Can also be used to measure Kyphosis and lordosis	

Power's Ratio

AB/CD
NL < 1.0

Skull Base

Anterior C1

Anterior C2

Anterior Humeral Line

Both lines should bisect central 1/3 of capitellum

Radio-Capitellar Line

Cobb Angle

Choose "end vertebra"; most tilted from the horizontal above the apex and below the apex of the curve. Draw a horizontal line across the upper end plate of the upper vertebra and the lower end plate of the lower vertebra. Draw a line perpendicular to these tangents until they intersect each other. The angle of the intersection is the Cobb angle.

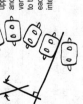

Scapholunate Angle
Nl 30 – 60°

Capitolunate angle
Nl < 30°

Osteoarthrosis V. Rheumatoid	
Osteophytes	None
Sclerosis	Osteopenia
Asymmetric	Symmetric
Subchondral cysts	Juxta-articular erosions

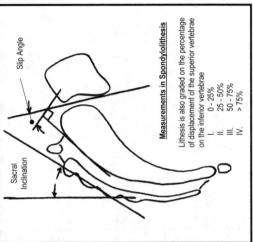

Measurements in Spondylolithesis

Lithesis is also graded on the percentage of displacement of the superior vertebrae on the inferior vertebrae

I.   0 - 25%
II.   25 - 50%
III. 50 - 75%
IV. >75%

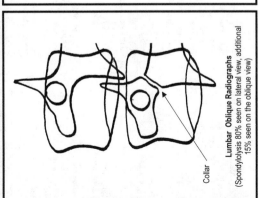

Lumbar Oblique Radiographs
(Spondylolysis 80% seen on lateral view, additional 15% seen on the oblique view)

Upper Extremity

LINE / ANGLE	NORMAL	DESCRIPTION	SIGNIFICANCE
Carrying Angle	10 - 20° 10 - 15° ♂ 15 - 20° ♀ 15° in kids	Angle formed by the longitudinal axis of the humerus and the longitudinal axis of the ulna measured in the frontal plane with the elbow in extension.	Carrying angle is usually symmetric and can be used as an indicator of malalignment
Anterior Humeral Line	Line passes through mid third of the lateral condylar ossific nucleus	Line carried straight down from the anterior cortex of the humeral diaphysis	Asymmetric, anterior, or posterior to the middle third of the capitellum indicative of fracture
Radio-Capitellar Line	Line passes thru mid 1/3 of capitellum	Line drawn down the longitudinal axis of the radius	Dislocation/subluxation of radial head (Monteggia fracture)
Wrist Arcs	Collinear	On lateral wrist, in neutral position, radial, lunate and capitate axes are co-linear. Seen on the PA radiograph of the wrist.	Asynchronous angulation indicative of carpal instability
Radio-lunate Angle (Lunate Tilt)	0°	Longitudinal axis of the radius with the axis of the lunate	> 15° flexion = VISI > 10° extension = DISI
Capito-lunate Angle	< 20°	Intersection of the capitate axis and lunate axis on the lateral wrist view	> 20° suggests carpal instability
Scapho-lunate Angle	30 – 60°	Angle formed by the scaphoid axis and the lunate axis	> 80° = DISI. ORIF scaphoid if > 60° and displaced > 1mm, < 30° = VISI
Scapholunate interval	< 3 mm	Gap between scaphoid and lunate on PA clenched fist view	Gap > 3 mm suggests scapholunate ligament tear, consider comparison view or dynamic study

VISI = Volar intercalated segmental instability, DISI = Dorsal intercalated segmental instability

Upper Extremity

LINE/ ANGLE	NORMAL	DESCRIPTION	SIGNIFICANCE
Radial Volar Tilt	11° volar (11 ± 2°)	On lateral view, angle formed by line drawn between the most distal volar and dorsal tips of the distal radius and a line drawn perpendicular to the longitudinal axis of the radius.	In fractures: >5mm of radial shortening on the PA or > 20° of dorsal angulation on the lateral is associated with a poor outcome.
Ulnar Variance	0 mm	On PA of wrist, draw one line perpendicular to the longitudinal axis of the radius and tangential to the articular pole of the distal ulna and one line perpendicular to the longitudinal axis of the radius and tangential to the lunate fossa of the distal radius. Measure the distance between the lines. Ulnar tangent distal to the radial tangent = positive ulnar variance.	0 mm = ulnar neutral, stress is distributed 80% to the proximal radius and 20% to the proximal ulna. + 4mm Ulnar positive variance the ratio is 60% ulna, 40% radius With negative ulnar variance the stress is 100% radius, 0% ulna.
Radial Inclination	22° (24 ± 2.5°)	The angle formed by the intersection of a line between the most distal points on the lateral and ulnar edges of the distal radius with a line perpendicular to the longitudinal axis of the radius on an PA view of the wrist	Useful in estimating the degree of deformity of distal radius fractures

MRI Signal Characteristics

T1 – fat, gadolinium, methemoglobin, proteinaceous fluid, melanoma
T2 – fluid
STIR – fluid (profoundly suppresses fat signal)
Gradient Echo – cartilage, "blooming" artifact in ferrous laden tissue (pigment villonodular synovitis)

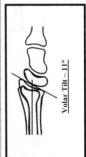

Volar Tilt ~ 11°

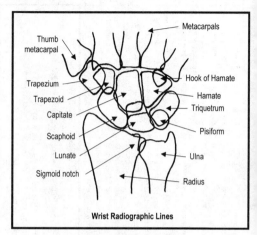

Wrist Radiographic Lines

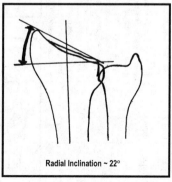

Radial Inclination ~ 22°

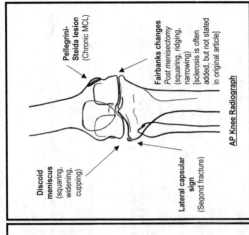

Pellegrini-Steida lesion (Chronic MCL)

Fairbanks changes
Post menisectomy (squaring, ridging, narrowing)
[sclerosis is often added, but not stated in original article]

Discoid meniscus (squaring, widening, cupping)

Lateral capsular sign (Segond fracture)

__AP Knee Radiograph__

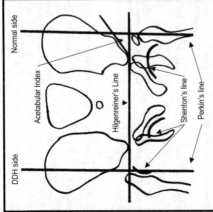

Normal side

DDH side

Acetabular Index

Hilgenreiner's Line

Shenton's line

Perkin's line

__DDH Lines and Radiographic Assessment__

Note: break in Shenton's line and absence of the ossific nucleus on DDH side

Hip/Pelvis

LINE / ANGLE	NORMAL	DESCRIPTION	SIGNIFICANCE
Perkins vertical line	Ossific nucleus medial to this line	A reference line that runs vertically through the lateral aspect of the bony acetabulum and is perpendicular to Hilgenreiner's line	Four quadrants are created by the intersection of Hilgenreiner's and Perkin's lines. In a subluxated hip, the femoral head will be in the lower, outer quadrant. In a dislocated hip, the femoral head is in the upper outer quadrant.
Hilgenreiner's line	Ossific nucleus inferior to this line	A horizontal reference line drawn through the triradiate cartilage	
Shenton's line (Curve)	Smooth curve without a break	Traces the arc between top of obturator foramen and medial femoral neck	Smooth curve broken in hip dysplasia, some fractures, and hip dislocation
Acetabular index	Birth < 30° 1 yr < 25° 3 yr < 20° 6 yr < 15° 10 yr < 10°	Angle formed a line drawn along the roof of the acetabulum and Hilgenreiner's Line	Indicates degree of acetabular dysplasia
Kline's line	Symmetric left-right	Line drawn tangent to the superior femoral neck on the AP pelvis	Can be suggestive of a SCFE (Warning – bilateral slips)
Epiphyseal angle	< 25°	Angle formed by a line tangent to proximal femoral epiphysis and Hilgenreiner's line	40 - 70° = Coxa Vara
Wiberg center edge angle (CE angle)	20 - 35° Abnormal = < 20°	Angle formed by a line drawn from center of the femoral head to the lateral edge of the acetabular roof and line through the center of the femoral head and perpendicular to Hilgenreiner's line	Decreased in dysplasia of the acetabulum as seen in hip dysplasia

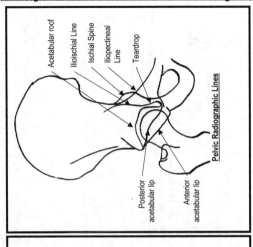

Acetabular roof
Ilioischial Line
Ischial Spine
Iliopectineal Line
Teardrop
Posterior acetabular lip
Anterior acetabular lip

Pelvic Radiographic Lines

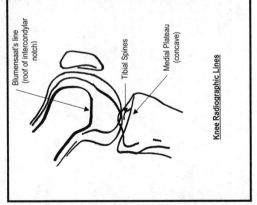

Blumensaat's line (roof of intercondylar notch)
Tibial Spines
Medial Plateau (concave)

Knee Radiographic Lines

Hip/Pelvis (Continued)

LINE /ANGLE	NORMAL	DESCRIPTION	SIGNIFICANCE
Neck shaft angle	124° ± 7°	Angle formed by a line drawn through the femoral neck and a line drawn through the femoral shaft	< 110° = Coxa vara of surgical significance. Coxa valga significance is variable, depends on acetabular coverage. Usually the ↑ the valgus the ↓ the coverage.
Iliopectineal line	No Cortical disruption	AP view. The most medial border of the pelvic ring. Oblique (obturator) View: the pelvic brim line, the anteromedial border of the anterior column	Cortical disruption indicates a fracture of the anterior column
Ilioischial line	No Cortical disruption	AP View of Pelvis: the serpiginous line that runs from the most distal juncture of the sacrum to the ischium, along the border of the ischium to the ischial tuberosity, and down to the distal juncture of the medial border of the posterior column of the acetabulum	Cortical disruption indicates a fracture of the posterior column. Teardrop may be 'V' or 'U' shaped in the presence of acetabular dysplasia.
Tear-drop	Tear drop shape; 5 - 8 mm medial to head > 5 - 8 mm suggests lateral displacement	AP hip/pelvis, teardrop shaped line medial to the head of the femur (quadrilateral plate)	Disruption suggests fracture or penetration through the acetabulum into the pelvis
Lower Extremity			
Q Angle	< 15°	Not a radiographic angle. Measured clinically from the angle derived by a line from the ASIS to the center of the patella, with a line from the center of the patella down the tibial spine.	Increased Q angle associated with laterally subluxated patella (from the increased lateral force of the quadriceps)

Lower Extremity

LINE /ANGLE	NORMAL	DESCRIPTION	SIGNIFICANCE
Proximal tibial metaphyseal-diaphyseal angle	< 11°	Angle formed by a line perpendicular to axis of the tibia and a line going through the medial and lateral lips of the proximal tibial metaphysis	In Varus, an angle > 11° suggests Blount's disease. Many feel > 14° = Blount's
Blumensaat's line	NA	A line drawn along the superior aspect of the intercondylar notch on a lateral knee view	The lower pole of the patella should reach this line. In patella alta, the lower pole is above this line
Insall ratio	1:1 Ratio	Measure on the lateral knee view flexed to 30°, ratio of patella length to length of patellar tendon	20% variation represents patella alta or patella baja
Sulcus angle	126 - 150° (average 138°)	Angle formed by a line drawn from the lowest point of intercondylar sulcus to highest points on the medial and lateral femoral condyles (Knee flexed 45° x-ray beam angled 30° from horizontal)	Larger angles are associated with subluxation or dislocation of the patella
Congruence angle	♂: -6° ♀: -10°	Angle formed by a line from apex of sulcus angle though lowest point of articular ridge of patella and line bisecting sulcus angle	Increased in patients with recurrent patella dislocations
Lateral patello-femoral angle (Laurin)	Opens laterally	Angle formed by a line drawn parallel to the lateral surface of the patella and a line drawn from the medial to lateral femoral condyles	Lines may be parallel or open medially in patients with recurrent patella subluxation

Foot/Ankle

LINE/ANGLE	NORMAL	DESCRIPTION	SIGNIFICANCE
Meary's angle	0°	Lateral foot x-ray: An angle formed by the longitudinal axis of the talus and the longitudinal axis of the first metatarsal	> 0° indicates cavus deformity due to forefoot cavus as opposed to hindfoot cavus
Gissane angle	120 - 145°	Angle that runs from the calcaneo-cuboid joint to the posterior margin of the posterior facet	May be altered in calcaneal fracture. It indicates the anterior, middle, and posterior facet relationships
Lateral talo-calcaneal angle	35 - 50°	Angle formed by a line drawn through the longitudinal axis of the talus and a line drawn along the plantar surface of the calcaneus	Decreased in club foot (Talipes Equinovarus)
Intermetatarsal angle	< 9°	Angle formed by lines through the longitudinal axis of the 1st and 2nd metatarsals	An angle of >15° merits consideration of a proximal osteotomy to correct deformity
First metatarsophalangeal angle	< 15°	Angle formed by a line through the longitudinal axis of the 1st metatarsal with that drawn through the longitudinal axis of the proximal phalanx	Increased in hallux valgus (bunions)
Anteroposterior talo-calcaneal angle (Kite's angle)	25 - 45°	An angle formed by the longitudinal axis of the calcaneus and the longitudinal axis of the talus	In club foot and hindfoot varus the angle is decreased. Approaches "parallelism"
Bohler's angle	25 - 40°	Measures the posterior facet height; shows degree of deformity and compression in calcaneal fractures	Angle may be increased, decreased, or reversed depending on the severity of the calcaneal fracture

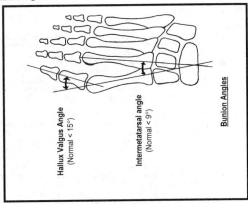

Hallux Valgus Angle
(Normal < 15°)

Intermetatarsal angle
(Normal < 9°)

Bunion Angles

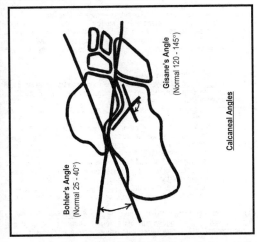

Bohler's Angle
(Normal 25 - 40°)

Gisane's Angle
(Normal 120 - 145°)

Calcaneal Angles

Sedation and Analgesia

Overview

Local anesthesia and blocks do not always provide the degree of analgesia optimal for performing many orthopaedic procedures. Associated anxiety and motion control can also be significant, especially in children. The goal of procedural sedation is to permit safe and effective control of pain, anxiety, and motion to enable a necessary procedure while providing an appropriate degree of amnesia or decreased awareness. Hospitals are required by the Joint Commission on Accreditation of Healthcare Organizations (JCAHO) to adhere to fairly strict requirements for any occurrence of procedural sedation in any location.

Sedation principles

- Sedation exists as a continuum from mild sedation/analgesia to general anesthesia (except for the dissociative agent ketamine).
- To best achieve a specified response on the sedation continuum, carefully titrate IV sedatives at spaced intervals (except for the dissociative agent ketamine).
- **Patients are at highest risk for developing complications during the 5-10 minutes following IV sedative administration and during the immediate post-procedure period when external stimuli are discontinued.**
- *Moderate sedation* (formerly "conscious sedation") is sedation to the point at which patients respond purposefully to verbal commands, either alone or accompanied by light tactile stimulation. No interventions are required to maintain a patent airway, and spontaneous ventilation is adequate.
- *Deep sedation* is more advanced than moderate sedation in that patients cannot be easily aroused, but still respond purposefully following repeated or painful stimulation. The ability to independently maintain ventilatory function may be impaired, and there is a higher risk of adverse events than with moderate sedation.

Sedation environment requirements

- <u>Resuscitation equipment</u>: oxygen, suction, age-appropriate bag-valve mask and intubation equipment. Reversal agents naloxone and flumazenil if opioids or benzodiazepines are being used, respectively.
- <u>Monitoring equipment</u>: continuous pulse oximetry, ECG monitoring, periodic vital signs as appropriate for sedation depth.
- <u>Personnel</u>: A minimum of two individuals experienced at procedural sedation: either two physicians, or one physician and one assistant (e.g., nurse, respiratory therapist). They must understand the pharmacology of their sedatives and be proficient at maintaining airway patency and assisting ventilation if needed. One individual must be available to continuously observe and monitor the patient for potential complications, although they may perform minor, interruptible assistant tasks. For deep or dissociative (i.e., ketamine) sedation one individual must have training in advanced life support interventions (e.g., airway management, resuscitation) and experience with this level of sedation.
- **<u>Pre-sedation evaluation</u>: Sedation must be preceded by a directed history and physical examination, with the following elements assessed *and documented* (JCAHO requirement): underlying medical problems**

(e.g., ASA physical status class), medications, allergies, previous adverse experience with sedation or general anesthesia, time and nature of last oral intake, heart & lung exam. The airway must be evaluated for abnormalities that might impair resuscitation.

- **Fasting:** For elective procedures, the American Society of Anesthesiologists recommends an age-stratified fasting guideline of 2 to 3 hours for clear liquids and 4 to 8 hours for solids and non-clear liquids. In non-fasting situations a risk-benefit analysis must be performed balancing the potential for vomiting and aspiration with the timing and urgency of the procedure and the required depth of sedation.
- **Discharge: Patients should be monitored until alert and oriented (or returned to age-appropriate baseline), and vital signs should be stable and at baseline.**

Sedation Drug Dosing (adapted from NEJM 2000; 342:938-945)*

Drug	Midazolam (*Versed*)	Fentanyl	Ketamine	Nitrous Oxide
Clinical effects	Sedation, motion control, anxiolysis. No analgesia. Reversible with flumazenil.	Analgesia. Reversible w/ naloxone.	Analgesia, dissociation, amnesia, motion control.	Mild anxiolysis, analgesia, sedation, amnesia
Adult dose	IV: Initial 1 mg, then titrated to max 5 mg. IM: 5 mg or 0.07 mg/kg IM	IV: 50 mcg, may repeat q3min, titrate	Not recommended; risk of unpleasant recovery reactions.	Preset mix with minimum 40% O₂ self-administered
Peds dose	IV (0.5-5 yrs): Initial 0.05-0.1 mg/kg, then titrated to max 0.6 mg/kg. IV (6-12 yrs): Initial 0.025-0.05 mg/kg, then titrated to max 0.4 mg/kg. IM: 0.1-0.15 mg/kg.	IV: 1.0 mcg/ kg/dose, repeat q3 min prn, titrate to effect	IV: 1-1.5 mg/kg slowly over 1-2 min, may repeat ½ dose q10min prn. IM: 4-5 mg/kg, may repeat after 10 min	by demand valve mask (requires cooperative patient)
Onset (min)	IV: 2-3 IM: 10-20	IV: 3-5	IV: 1 IM: 3-5	<5
Duration (min)	IV: 45-60 IM: 60-120	IV: 30-60	IV: dissociation 15; recovery 60. IM: diss 15-30; rec 90-150	<5 minutes following discontinuation
Comments	Reduce dose when used in combination with opioids. May produce paradoxical excitement.	Reduce dosing when combined with midazolam	Multiple contraindications, administer concurrent atropine to prevent hypersalivation. mg/kg, min. 0.1 mg, max. 0.5 mg	Requires gas scavenging & special equip. Several contraindications

*Alterations in dosing may be indicated based upon the clinical situation & the practitioner's experience with these agents. Doses may vary when used in combination with other agents, especially when benzodiazepines are combined with opioids. Use lower doses in geriatric patients and those with significant cardiopulmonary disease.

References: McCarty: Ketamine sedation for the reduction of children's fractures in the ED. *J Bone Joint Surg* 2000; 7:912-918. Krauss: Sedation & analgesia for procedures in children. *N Engl J Med* 2000; 342:938-945. JCAHO: www.jacho.org/standard/aneshap.html ASA: Practice guidelines for sedation & analgesia by non-anesthesiologists. *Anesthesiology* 1996; 84:459-471.

Concussions In Athletes (Observe and evaluate for at least 15 minutes)[48]

Grade	Symptoms	Duration	Recommended return
1	Confusion, no amnesia	Minutes	When symptoms resolve
2	Retrograde amnesia	Hours to days	1 week*
3	Amnesia after impact	Days	1 month*

*Second episode - out for the entire season.

Any athlete that is symptomatic after a concussion requires serial evaluation.

If at any point exam reveals deterioration in mental status or loss of consciousness after a concussion immediate transportation to an emergency facility is indicated.

Return to Play Criteria

Same Day	Not the same day
Signs and symptoms cleared in 15 minutes	Signs and symptoms last >15 min
Normal neurologic examination	
No documented loss of consciousness	Signs and symptoms return
	Documented loss of consciousness
Any new headache within 48 - 72 hours - No play, full medical evaluation	
Beware unilateral headache in the younger athlete	

Significant signs and symptoms
Dizziness, slowness to respond, difficulty concentrating, physical sluggishness, memory loss (especially retrograde)

Post concussion syndrome (occurs with grade 2/3)
Persistent headaches, irritability, confusion, difficulty concentrating

Classic concussion
Includes an unconscious period. (> 5 minutes obtain CT)

Diffuse axonal injury
Defined by LOC > 6 hr - consider avoidance of all future contact sports

Steroids in Emergent Cord Injury[49]	
Contraindications: Age < 13 (controversial), nerve root or cauda equina, gunshot wounds, pregnancy, already on steroids, other life threatening injury.	
Therapy (Methylprednisone) initiated within	
3 hours after injury:	From 3 - 8 hours after injury:
30 mg/kg IV for the first hour	30 mg/kg IV for the first hour
5.4 mg/kg/hr IV for the next 23 hours	5.4 mg/kg/hr IV for the next 47 hours

Autonomic Dysreflexia
Catastrophic hypertensive event caused by impacted feces or an obstructed urinary catheter and occurs with complete spinal cord injury above T8 - T10.

---

48 Wojtys EM, et al. Concussion in Sports. Am J Sports Med 1999;27:5 676-685.
49 Bracken NEJM 1997;277:1597

Spondylolysis and Spondylolithesis

Class	Type	Age	Pathology/Other
I	Congenital	Child	Dysplastic S1 superior facet
II	Isthmic	5 - 50	Elongation/fracture of L5 S1 pars
III	Degenerative	Older	Subluxation due to facet (L4 L5) arthrosis
IV	Traumatic	Young	Acute fracture (not pars)
V	Pathologic	Any	Bony elements destroyed/incompetent
VI	Post surgical	Adult	Over resected arches/facets

Lithesis Grades	Spondylolysis
I. 0 - 25%	Defect in the pars interarticularis
II. 25 - 50%	Most common cause of low back pain in children
III. 50 - 75%	Fatigue fracture (gymnastics, football linemen)
IV. 75 - 100%	80% visible on plain films, 15% on obliques (Scottie Dog)
V. >100%	Treatment is symptomatic, avoid extension
	Casting for more severe or symptomatic cases

Muscle Strength Testing	
Score	Exam
0	No movement
1	Visible contraction
2	Movement without gravity
3	Movement with gravity
4	Less than full strength
5	Full strength

Reflexes	
Root Level	Reflex
C5	Biceps
C6	Brachioradialis
C7	Triceps
L4	Knee jerk
S1	Ankle jerk

Frankel Grade	
Grade	Function
A	Complete Paralysis
B	Sensory Function only below level of injury
C	Incomplete motor function (grade 1-2/5) below injury level
D	Fair to good motor function (grade 3-4/5) below injury level
E	Normal function (5/5)

Upper v. Lower Motor Lesions[50]		
Findings	UMN	LMN
Strength	↓	↓
Tone	↑	↓
Deep tendon reflex	↑	↓
Superficial tendon reflex	↓	↓
Babinski	+	-
Clonus	+	-
Fasciculations	-	+
Atrophy	-	+

[50] Simon SR. Orthopedic Basic Science, 2nd ed. page 354,Rosemont, IL AAOS, 1994.

Spinal Cross Section

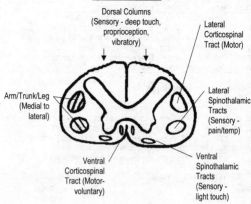

Dorsal Columns
(Sensory - deep touch,
proprioception,
vibratory)

Lateral
Corticospinal
Tract (Motor)

Arm/Trunk/Leg
(Medial to
lateral)

Lateral
Spinothalamic
Tracts (Sensory -
pain/temp)

Ventral
Corticospinal
Tract (Motor-
voluntary)

Ventral
Spinothalamic
Tracts (Sensory -
light touch)

Low Back Pain Red Flags

Trauma	Demonstrable muscle weakness
> 50 years old	Bowel or bladder dysfunction/incontinence
Fever	Saddle anesthesia
History of cancer	Decreased sphincter tone
Metabolic disorder	Night pain
	Unexplained weight loss

Low Back Pain Treatment

Acute LBP (≤ 6 weeks)
70% better in 2 wks, 90% better in 4 - 6 weeks
-NSAIDS or acetaminophen (Opiates/muscle relaxants of no additional benefit)
-Minimize bedrest (encourage modified light activity)
-Radiographs or MRI in the presence of red flags

Chronic LBP (>6 weeks), Worsening radiculopathy
-Rule out cauda equina syndrome - surgical emergency
-Radiographs, MRI as indicated
-Enlist the aid of pain clinic, mental health, etc.
**Workman's compensation and litigation have worse long term prognosis

Spinal Cord injury Syndromes

SYNDROME	Mechanism of Injury/Pathology	Characteristics	Prognosis
Central	Age > 50, extension injury, ? vascular etiology	Upper > lower extremities, motor and sensory loss	Fair
Anterior	Flexion-Compression	Incomplete motor, some sensory loss	Poor
Brown-Sequard	Penetrating trauma	Loss of ipsilateral motor, contralateral pain and temperature	Best
Root	Foraminal Compression/ Herniated disc	Based on level	Good
Complete	Burst fracture, canal compromise	No function below level of injury	Poor

Adapted from Miller MD (ed.): Review of Orthopaedics, 3rd ed. Philadelphia, WB Saunders, 2000, page 358, with permission

Spinal Cord Injury Treatment by Functional Level

Level	Working	Not Working	Treatment/Mobility
<C4	-	Diaphragm, Upper extremities	Respirator dependent
C4	Diaphragm/Trapezius	Upper extremities	Wheelchair chin/puff
C5	**Elbow Flexors**	Below Elbow	**Electric Wheelchair, ratchet**
C6	Wrist Extensors	Elbow extensors	Wheelchair, flexor hinge
C7	**Elbow Extensors**	Grasp	**Wheelchair, independent**
T1	Intrinsics	Abdominals, Lower extremities	Wheelchair, independent
T2-12	Upper extremities, abdominals	Lower extremities	Wheelchair, HKAFO (non functional ambulation)
L1	Upper extremities, abdominals, Quads	Lower extremities	KAFO, Minimal ambulation
L2	Iliopsoas	Knee/ankle	KAFO, household ambulation
L3	**Quadriceps**	Ankle	**AFO, Community amb.**
L4	Tibialis anterior	Toe dorsi flexion, plantar flexors	AFO, Community ambulation
L5	Extensor Hallucis & Digitorum Longus	Plantar flexors	AFO, Independent
S1	Gastrocnemius, Soleus	Bowel/Bladder	± Metatarsal bar

Level = Functional level, Functional level is the most distal intact motor level (fair motor grade). HKAFO hip knee ankle foot orthosis, KAFO knee ankle foot orthosis, AFO ankle foot orthosis
Adapted from Miller MD (ed.): Review of Orthopaedics, 3rd ed. Philadelphia, WB Saunders, 2000, page 458, with permission

Traction set-ups[51]

General Principles-
- Skin traction should not be used over an open wound.
- Skin traction should not be used when it would impede or affect the neuro-vascular status of the limb.
- Ensure no history of allergies to skin adhesives.
- Do not re-use traction cord.
- Pad all bony prominences.
- All weights must hang free and must not lie above the patient.
- Knots must be free from pulleys, especially in dynamic traction.
- Likewise, the moving parts of the traction set up should be free from interference from bed, bed sheets, etc.
- You must communicate and explain the basic principles and dangers to the support staff.
- Patient transport should be done under physician supervision, or the traction set up rechecked upon arrival at any new location.
- Skin care and neurovascular status need to be monitored regularly.

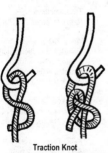

Traction Knot
(Up and over, down and over, up and through)
Leaving 10 cm at the end of the cord allows for fine adjustment throughout the course of traction.

Traction Pin Placement

Calcaneal Traction Pin
The pin is placed on the bone via a incision through the skin and blunt dissection down to the calcaneus. It is placed from **medial to lateral**. The pin is positioned at a point 2.5 cm inferior and 2.5 cm posterior to the tip of the lateral malleolus on the medial aspect of the calcaneus. The pin is then drilled through the calcaneus and delivered via a stab incision laterally. Care is taken to protect the medial neurovascular structures and the subtalar joint.

TRACTION IS NOT BENIGN!

51 Zimmer Traction Handbook: A Complete Reference Guide to the Basics of Traction. Zimmer, Inc. 1992.

Distal femoral pin

-90-90 position placed **medial to lateral**
-Parallel to the joint surface
-90 degrees to the shaft
-5/64 or 3/32 - threaded Steinmann pin, when the pin
  tents the lateral skin an incision is used to deliver it
  through the skin.
-Pin level is 1 fingerbreadth above patella with the
  knee extended or just above the distal femoral
  flare.
-If intramedullary fixation is planned the pin must be
  placed anterior or posterior to the center to allow
  for rod passage.
-Pin is passed **medial to lateral** to protect
  neurovascular structures through Hunters canal
  (adductor hiatus)

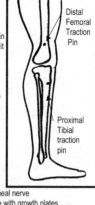

Distal Femoral Traction Pin

Proximal Tibial traction pin

Proximal Tibial traction pin

-At the level of the tibial tubercle
-1-2 cm posterior to anterior tibial crest
-Passed **lateral to medial** to protect common peroneal nerve
-Not favored in children due to potential interference with growth plates

Traction Types

Pediatric Traction

-In general skeletal traction is not recommended as a method of treatment for
  children over 12 years old (increased incidence of shortening and angulation)
-Indications include unstable femur fracture < 6 years old, > 3 cm shortening; femur
  fracture < 6 years old, unstable in hip spica; associated other injuries in a child
  able to cooperate with bed rest.
-Skin complications can occur with > 5 pounds skin traction.

Bryant's Traction (rarely used, NV complications)

-Hips at 90°, knees at 0°, Chest restraint, Bradford frame, Weight adjusted to just
  lift the sacrum off the Bradford frame
  (do not use in > 2 years, > 25 lb., Beware of serious neurovascular compromise)

Modified Bryant's Traction

-Decreases incidence of neurovascular compromise.
-May use in older patients with contraindications to a femoral traction pin.

Russell Skin Traction /Split Russell's Traction (adults and children)

-Peroneal nerve neuropraxia possible.
-Posterior bowing at fracture site possible

Bucks Traction

-Elevate the foot of the bed, Closely monitor skin!

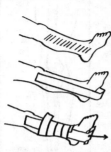

Application of Skin Traction
Benzoin to lateral and medial leg.
Horseshoe of adhesive backed felt.
Wrap loosely with an Ace wrap.
Include metal traction bar in felt loop.

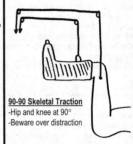

90-90 Skeletal Traction
-Hip and knee at 90°
-Beware over distraction

**Distal Femoral traction pin is placed
with the knee flexed so the iliotibial band
does not drag over the pin

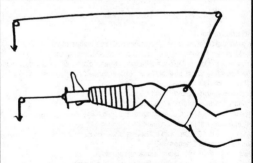

Russell's Skin Traction
Skin traction of leg
Pillow or traction set-up supporting femur
Sling may also be placed on leg with a pillow supporting the thigh

Lateral Arm Traction
(lateral and overhead)

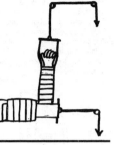

-Elbow at 90° of flexion
-Shoulder at 90° of abduction, neutral
  flexion/extension
-Traction to humerus only, forearm weights
  only for neutralization of forearm weight

Lateral Arm Traction Set-up ➡

Balanced Suspension (with/without skeletal traction)
-Elevate foot of bed

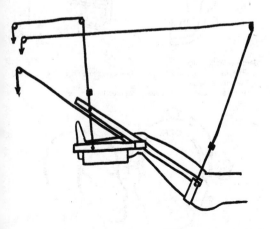

Halo Placement

-Halo is placed just below the area of greatest circumference, just above the eyebrows, and ~ 1cm above ear tips.
-Pins placed with local anesthetic, positions as shown.
-Eyes closed tightly. Areas shaved.
-Pins subsequently tightened circumferentially in a diagonal, opposite manner. 2 lb.-in, 4 lb.-in., and finally 6 - 8 lb.-in (adults) 4 - 6 lb.-in. (child <5yo), 2 lb.-in. or finger tight in infants/toddlers. Children need multiple pins (up to 8).
-Retighten at 24 - 48 hr.

Medial to lateral
1. Frontal sinus
2. Supratrochlear n.
3. Supraorbital n.

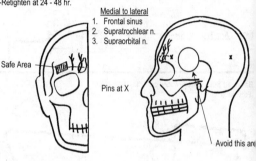

Safe Area

Pins at X

Avoid this are

Gardener-Wells Tongs

-Pins positioned below the temporal ridges, 2 cm above ext. auditory canal and temporalis muscle.
-Tongs are secure when pressure pin extrudes 1 mm.

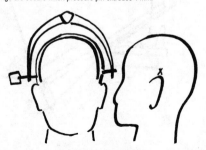

Hand

Injury/Eponym	Classification	Treatment
Distal phalanx fracture	Longitudinal, transverse, comminuted	Splint 3-4 weeks, > 50% nailbed hematoma – fix nailbed
Extensor digitorum avulsion (terminal tendon) *Mallet finger*	Stretched	Splint distal interphalangeal joint in extension
	Torn	Full time for 6 weeks
	Bony avulsion	Then only at night for 4-6 weeks
FDP avulsion *Rugger Jersey Finger*	Leddy/Packer	
	I – tendon retracts to palm	Fix within 7-10 days
	II – tendon retracts to PIPJ	Fix within 2 weeks (may repair late up to 3 months)
	III – bony fragment retracts to A4 pulley	ORIF (early)
	IIIA (IV) – bony fragment & avulsed tendon	ORIF & reattach tendon (early)
Metacarpal and Phalangeal fracture.	Indications for operative treatment	Goal – Full & rapid restoration of function!
	-Malrotation (spiral, oblique)	Dealers (surgeons) choice
	-Intraarticular, -Open fracture (relative)	-ORIF (associated with stiffness)
	-Sub capital phalangeal fracture	-Open reduction, percutaneous pinning
	-Bone loss, -Polytrauma & hand fracture	-Closed reduction, percutaneous pinning
	-Multiple hand/wrist fractures	-Traction [used uncommonly – PIPJ fracture/dislocations]
	-Fracture with soft tissue injury	-ORIF (Composite wiring, intramedullary fixation, external
	-Reconstruction	fixation)
Central slip disruption *Boutonniere*	Soft tissue	Acute or chronic –
	Bony fragment	Extension splint x 6 weeks
		(flexion contracture corrects slowly)
Extensor tendon laceration	< 50% laceration	Primary closure, rehabilitation
	> 50% laceration	Repair tendon, rehabilitation
Flexor tendon laceration	Zone specific classification (See page 90)	Tendon repair may delay up to 2 - 3 weeks, atraumatic technique, strict supervised rehabilitation post operatively

Hand (Continued)

Injury/Eponym	Classification	Treatment
4th/5th metacarpal neck *Boxers fracture*	20 - 45° angulation acceptable Check rotation!	Closed reduction cast/splint x 3 - 4 weeks
2nd/3rd metacarpal neck	15° is acceptable	Percutaneous pinning to adjacent metacarpal or ORIF
Transverse metacarpal	Accept 50 - 70° 4th & 5th, 20° 2nd & 3rd	Closed reduction/cast versus ORIF
Oblique metacarpal	< 5mm short	Closed reduction or open reduction, percutaneous pinning
	> 5mm or malrotation	ORIF
Thumb metacarpal *Bennett's* →	intra-articular volar lip	Closed reduction, percutaneous pinning, ORIF if necessary
Rolando's →	intra-articular Y	ORIF (if non-comminuted)
		External fixation/traction (if comminuted)
	transverse	Closed reduction spica cast x 4 week
	oblique	Closed reduction spica cast x 4 week
5th MC base		Most stable (if not)
Baby Bennett	Intraarticular base fracture	Closed reduction, percutaneous pinning

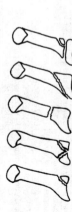

Boutonniere – Note central slip disruption, volar subluxation of lateral bands, characteristic deformity, tenderness over PIPJ may be only obvious clinical sign

Bennett's   Rolando's   Transverse   Oblique   Salter-Harris II

Hand (Continued)

Injury/Eponym	Classification	Treatment
DIPJ dislocation	Dorsal	Closed reduction, splint x 2 weeks
	With collateral sprain	Buddy tape 3 - 6 weeks
	With collateral tear	Fix radial collateral ligament (index, ring, and middle)
		Fix ulnar collateral ligament (small finger, dominant hand)
Dorsal PIPJ dislocation	Dorsal (volar plate torn)	Closed reduction (open if not reducible)
	I - Hyper extension	Buddy tape or extension block splint
	II - Major ligament injury	Extension block splint
	III - Proximal dislocation	> 4 mm displacement – ORIF, congruous – extension splint x 4-6 wk
Volar PIPJ dislocation	Volar (central slip torn)	ORIF irreducible or incongruous
	Rotatory	Attempted closed reduction, open if fails closed reduction
Dorsal PIPJ fracture-disloc.	Located	Extension block
	Subluxated ("V" sign dorsally - Light)	Volar plate arthroplasty, ORIF, traction splint, force couple pinning
MCPJ dislocation	Collateral ligament injury	Splint MCP 50° x 3 weeks, ORIF > 2 - 3 mm or > 20% joint surface
	Dorsal	
	-Simple	Closed reduction, splint x 7-10 days
	-Complex (Volar plate interposition)	Open reduction
	Volar	Open reduction (sesamoid in ↑ joint space, skin puckered palmar, less deformity seen)
CMCJ dislocation	Small finger CMCJ dislocation	Closed reduction, percutaneous pinning
	Multiple CMCJ dislocation	Open reduction, percutaneous pinning
Thumb MCPJ ulnar collateral ligament injury	Sprain (<35° on stress views)	Thumb spica cast x 6 weeks
	Tear (> 35°)	Open repair
Gamekeeper	(Steiner lesion = adductor aponeurosis interposition between torn ends)	

Hand (Continued)

Injury/Eponym	Classification	Treatment
Thumb MCPJ radial collateral ligament	Sprain/tear	Splint, percutaneous pinning
Thumb MCPJ dorsal dislocation	Simple	Reduce, cast x 3 weeks
	Complex	Single reduction attempt, (Volar plate ± Flexor pollicus longus interposition)
Thumb CMCJ dislocation		Hyper pronation & percutaneous pinning Cast 6 - 10 weeks
Hamate metacarpal fracture/ dislocation	Cain	
	IA-ligament injury	reduce/stable-cast, reduce/unstable-percutaneous pinning
	IB-dorsal hamate fracture	reduce/stable-cast, reduce/unstable-ORIF
	II-comminuted dorsal hamate fracture	ORIF-restore dorsal buttress
	III-coronal hamate fracture	ORIF-restore joint surface (GOAL: < 2 mm step off, < 5mm short)

Wrist

Injury/Eponym	Classification	Treatment
Distal radius Colle's (dorsal) Smith's (volar)	No single classification	
	Extra articular	Closed reduction, cast External fixation, bone graft, and/or ORIF (higher energy, older bone, significant displacement.)
	Intraarticular	Restore joint surface
Dorsal rim distal radius Dorsal Barton's		Reduce, pronation ORIF if necessary
Radial styloid – Chauffeur's		Reduce, percutaneous pinning or cannulated screw, cast in ulnar deviation
Volar rim - Volar Barton's		ORIF

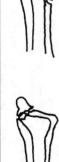

Dorsal Barton's   Volar Barton's   Radial Styloid

Wrist (Continued)

Injury/Eponym	Classification	Treatment
Distal Radio Ulnar Joint	Dorsal	Reduce, long arm cast in supination x 6 weeks
	Volar	Reduce, long arm cast in pronation x 6 weeks
		Open reduction ± internal fixation if irreducible
Scaphoid	Can be classified based on time or anatomic configuration	Stable/non-displaced- long arm cast up to 3+ months
		Unstable/displaced [1 mm, scapholunate > 60°, lunatocapitate > 15°] – ORIF
[blood supply dorsal and distal]		
Dorsal chip	Commonly triquetrum	Short arm cast x 6 weeks
Hook of Hamate	CT to evaluate	Excise for persistent pain
Perilunate dislocation ± scaphoid fracture	Mayfield (stage II = I + II, III = II + III, etc.)	Early (6 - 8 weeks)-
	I - Scapholunate dissociation	Open reduction, ligament repair, percutaneous pinning.
	II - Lunocapitate dissociation	ORIF scaphoid fracture if present
	III - Lunotriquetral disruption	
	IV - Lunate dislocation	

Radius/Ulnar Shaft

Radius and ulna – *Both bone*	Non-displaced or displaced	ORIF

Radius/Ulnar Shaft (Continued)

Injury/Eponym	Classification	Treatment
Ulna fracture	Non-displaced	Long arm cast or fracture brace (accept 10° and 50% displacement)
Nightstick	Displaced	ORIF - beware wrist/elbow injury
Proximal ulna fracture/ radial head dislocation	*Bado*	
Monteggia	I - radial head anterior	ORIF, closed reduction head
	II - head posterior	
	III - head lateral	
	IV - head anterior & both bone fracture	
Proximal Radius	Non-displaced	Long arm cast in supination, close follow up
	Displaced	ORIF
Distal radius fracture & radio-ulnar dissociation	*Eponyms - Galeazzi, Piedmont, Reverse Monteggia, fracture of necessity, etc.*	

Elbow

Supra-condylar	Extension	
Malgaigne	-Non-displaced	Long arm cast
	-Displaced	ORIF (double plating)
Trans-condylar	(very uncommon fracture)	
Kocher	Intra articular – posterior fragment	Reduce (closed treatment difficult, ankylosis common), percutaneous pinning, ORIF if necessary (no consensus in the literature)
Posadas	Intra articular – anterior fragment	
Condylar	I - Lateral trochlear ridge intact	Non-displaced – long arm cast in supination (lateral), long arm cast in pronation (medial), some need ORIF
Milch (lateral >medial)	II - Fracture through lateral trochlear ridge	ORIF

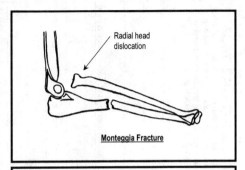

Mont[e]ggia Fracture

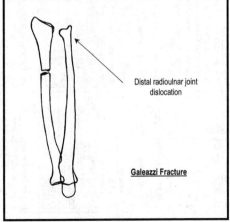

Galeazzi Fracture

Elbow (Continued)

Injury/Eponym	Classification	Treatment

Bicolumnar	Jupiter (see page 133)
	1 - T
	  (a. high, b. low)
	2 - Y
	3 - H
	4 - Lambda
	  (a. medial, b. lateral)
		Generally these fractures are treated operatively. Restoration of the joint surface is paramount. Rigid fixation with early motion (immobilize < 2 weeks) helps to avoid fibrosis/ankylosis that occurs with prolonged immobilization. Total elbow replacement may be considered in the elderly with osteoporotic bone where fixation may be difficult or impossible to attain.

Olecranon	Cotton I - Non displaced II - Displaced A - Avulsion B - Oblique/ transverse C - Comminuted D - Fracture/dislocation	Cast/splint, 3 weeks or less ORIF (tension band) Oblique - screw Transverse - tension band Excise (coronoid and anterior structures must be intact, reattach triceps to bone) ORIF (no excision)
Coronoid	Regan/Morrey I - tip avulsion II - < 50% III - > 50%	Early motion Early motion ORIF
Capitellar Hahn-Steinthal Kocher-Lorenz	I - large trochlear piece II - minimal subchondral bone (Kocher-LoRENZ sounds like lens) III - comminuted (rare)	Non-displaced-splint, Displaced-ORIF Non-displaced-splint Displaced-ORIF versus excise ORIF versus excision

Elbow (Continued)

Injury/Eponym	Classification	Treatment
Trochlea *Laugier*	Very rare	Non-displaced - splint Displaced -ORIF
Epicondylar	Medial (*Granger*) more common than lateral	Manipulation/reduction, posterior splint with the elbow and wrist flexed x 10 – 14 days, then active motion is begun, symptomatic fragments can be excised late

High T   Low T   Y Type

H Type   Medial Lambda   Lateral Lambda

Hahn-Steinthall   Kocher-Lorenz

Elbow (Continued)

Injury/Eponym	Classification	Treatment
Radial Head	Mason I - Non displaced	Early motion, ± aspiration
	II - Moderate displacement	Treat like type I for no mechanical block, ORIF for mechanical block, or consider ORIF if ± 1/3 of joint, >30° angulation, > 3mm stepoff
	III - Comminuted	ORIF versus excision
	IV - With dislocation	Reduce dislocation, ORIF
Elbow dislocation	General principles	Stable- closed reduction, < 7days immobilize, Unstable- open repair.
	Types – Posterior (commonest 90%)	Humeral countertraction, distal forearm traction, correct medial/lateral 1st, then distal traction and flexion
	Anterior	Reversal of posterior technique
	Medial/lateral	Humeral countertraction, distal forearm traction, medial/lateral slide
	Divergent	Reduce ulna 1st, radius 2nd

Shoulder

Injury/Eponym	Classification	Treatment
Humeral shaft	Location/Pattern [Spiral & radial nerve injury = Holstein-Lewis]	Coaptation splint, cast brace, or hanging arm cast. ORIF- floating elbow, segmental, pathologic, obesity, ipsilateral chest wall injury, poly trauma, bilateral fractures, or unacceptable alignment in splint (> 30° varus/valgus, > 20° anterior/posterior, > 3 cm short, or radial nerve palsy post reduction).
Proximal Humerus	Neer 1 part	Early motion
	2 part	Closed reduction
(A part is defined as > 1 cm displaced or > 45° angulated)		ORIF (articular segment)
		Cuff repair ± closed reduction & fixation– Greater tuberosity
	3 part	ORIF (Hemiarthroplasty-elderly)
	4 part	Prosthesis (prosthesis also indicated for a head splitting fracture)

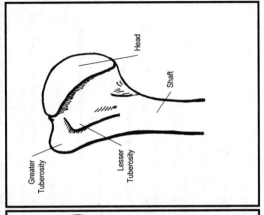

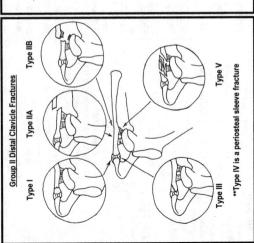

Shoulder (Continued)

Injury/ Eponym	Classification	Treatment
Proximal humerus fracture/ dislocation	Anterior (Greater Tuberosity displaced)	5 mm post reduction – ORIF
	Posterior (Lesser Tuberosity displaced)	Closed reduction, ORIF if 3 part
Impression	Stable (<20%)	Closed treatment
Hill-Sachs	Unstable (20-50%)	Transfer lesser tuberosity to defect
	(>50%)	Prosthesis versus osteotomy
Head Splitting		Prosthesis
Clavicle	Group I: Middle 1/3 (85%)	Group I: Majority heal with non-operative treatment
	Group II: (see page 135) Distal 1/3 (Neer) (10%) I - Minimal displacement II - Medial to Coraco-clavicular ligament A - Ligaments intact & with distal fragment B - Conoid torn, trapezoid with intact distal fragment III - Involving acromioclavicular joint IV - Periosteal sleeve V - Comminuted	Group II: I & IV - Conservative IIA & IIB & V - ORIF III-Closed treatment, late acromioclavicular excision for arthrosis
		Group III: Non-operative
	Group III: Medial 1/3 (5%)	Group I & III: ORIF - open fracture, displaced with skin compromise, associated with vascular injuries needing repair

Shoulder Girdle (Cont.)

Injury/Eponym	Classification	Treatment
Scapula	Zdravkovich & Damholt	
	I - Body	Closed treatment
	II - Coracoid & acromion	ORIF large displaced fragment (associated injury common)
	III - Neck & tubercle	ORIF large displaced fragment
Glenoid	Ideberg	
	I - Anterior avulsion	ORIF if > 25% glenoid involved and humeral head subluxated
	II - Transverse/oblique fracture inferior glenoid free	
	III - Upper 1/3 glenoid & coracoid	
	IV - Horizontal glenoid thru body	
	V - Combination II-IV	
Scapulothoracic dissociation	Internal forequarter amputation	Closed reduction, massive internal trauma, massive vascular & brachial plexus injuries
Anterior dislocation	Subcoracoid > subglenoid	Reduce: <u>Stimson</u> – prone, arm hanging with weight at wrist <u>Milch</u> – external rotation, abduction, posteriorly directed force on the anterior of the shoulder Traction/countertraction – stabilize chest, distal/abduction traction on forearm, add gentle rotation Confirm reduction (x-rays), immobilize (classically comfortable adduction/internal rotation)
Posterior dislocation	Seizure, electrical shock	Lateral upper arm traction, distal lower arm traction & gentle rotation
Inferior dislocation	*Luxatio erecta*	Reduce/immobilize

Shoulder Girdle (Cont.)

Injury/Eponym	Classification	Treatment
Rotator cuff tear	Partial	Rehabilitation, debride if fails conservative
	Complete	Rehabilitation, surgical repair in athletes, failed conservative treatment
Acromio-clavicular injury (percent displaced in [ ])	I - Acromioclavicular ligament (AC) sprain [0%]	Sling/range of motion
	II - AC tear, coracoclavicular (CC) sprain [0 -25%]	Sling/range of motion
	III - AC, CC [25 - 100%]	Selective ORIF (not in contact sports)
	IV - Clavicular subluxated posterior into trapezius	Reduce/repair
	V - Type III with large displacement [100-300%]	Reduce/repair
	VI - Clavicle suboracoid	Reduce/repair
Sternoclavicular injury	Anterior	Closed reduction with traction
	Posterior	Closed reduction with towel clip, open reduction if closed reduction fails (beware great vessels, thoracic surgeon available)
	Atraumatic	Non-operative
Biceps Tendon	Distal	Surgical repair
	Proximal	Rehabilitation
Cervical Spine		
Occipital condyle fracture	Anderson/Montesano	
	I - Impaction	Hard collar
	II - Plus skull fracture	Hard collar
	III - Avulsion	May require halo immmobilization

Cervical Spine (Continued)

Injury/Eponym	Classification	Treatment
Occiput-C1 Dislocation	Anterior or posterior (usually fatal)	Halo & occiput/C1 fusion
C1 Fracture (*Jefferson* = axial load)	Symmetric axial compression (fracture of ring in 3 - 4 places, lateral masses forced apart)	Stable fractures (posterior arch or non displaced fractures) treated with cervical orthosis
	Asymmetric axial force (isolated lateral mass Displacement)	Asymmetric lateral mass fracture or Jefferson "burst" fractures require halo immobilization
	Hyperextension (posterior arch fracture)	Transverse ligament rupture without a bony avulsion requires fusion
Odontoid fracture	**Anderson/ D'Alonzo**	
	I - Oblique apical/ avulsion	Cervical orthosis (beware associated injury)
	II - Base fracture	Halo vest, internal fixation for age > 50, > 5 mm, displaced posterior displacement, – screw fixation versus fusion
	III - Fracture into body	Halo immobilization
Traumatic spondylolisthesis of C2 *Hangman's*	**Levine**	
	I - Non-displaced (No angulation, < 3 mm)	Cervical orthosis
	II - Displaced/angulated	Reduction/halo
	IIa - C2 - 3 disc torn, anterior longitudinal ligament intact	Reduction/halo
	III - Fracture/ dislocation	Attempt reduction (< 4 mm translation, < 10° angulation) halo (failure - rule out disc rupture, ± fusion)
C3-C7 Facet dislocation	Unilateral (< 25% displacement of vertebral body) Bilateral (25 - 50% displacement of vertebral body)	Traction (10 lb + 5 lb/level), open reduction/ posterior fusion failed closed reduction, consider MRI rule out disc herniation

Cervical Spine (Continued)

Injury/Eponym	Classification	Treatment
C3-C7 Fracture	Translation	> 3.5 mm - fusion
	Angular displacement	> 11° - fusion
C3-C7 Burst	Canal Compression	< 25% compression with intact posterior wall = non-operative, Stable = Halo immobilization, unstable = fusion
C3-7 Spinous process fracture	*Clay Shovelers*	Symptomatic

Thoracic and Lumbar Spine

Injury/Eponym	Classification	Treatment
Burst fracture	A - Axial load B - Axial & flexion C - Axial & flexion D - Axial & rotation E - Axial & lateral flexion	Stable = hyperextension cast/brace Unstable (height <50%, angulation >20°, canal compromise > 50%, scoliosis > 10°, neurologic injury) = early operative stabilization
Flexion/ distraction		Bony = hyperextension cast
Chance		Soft tissue = ORIF
Fracture -dislocation	Flexion - rotation Shear	ORIF = early mobilization

Clinical Instability in the Lower Cervical Spine[52]

2 points each – Anterior elements destroyed or functionless, posterior elements destroyed or functionless, sagittal plane translation >3.5mm, relative sagittal plane rotation >11°, positive stretch test, spinal cord damage

1 point each – Nerve root damage, abnormal disc narrowing, dangerous loading anticipated

> 5 is unstable

[52] White AA, Southwick WO, Panjabi MM. Clinical instability in the lower cervical spine: A review of past and current concepts. Spine1:15, 1976.

Fracture types and Columnar involvement[53]

Type	Anterior	Middle	Posterior
Compression	Compression	None	None or distraction
Burst	Compression	Compression	None or distraction
Seat-belt	None or compression	Distraction	Distraction
Fracture/dislocation	Compression ± rotation/shear	Distraction ± rotation/shear	Distraction ± rotation/shear

Pelvis Fractures

Injury/Eponym	Classification	Treatment
Pelvis (see page 142)	**Young & Burgess**	(See algorithm page 142)
LC = Lateral Compression	Lateral compression (LC) I - Sacral compression, transverse anterior ring injury (fracture versus symphysis injury)	Non weight bearing, selected stabilization
	LCII - Sacral/iliac wing fracture, anterior ring fracture (sacrospinous (SS) & sacrotuberous (ST) ligament intact)	External fixation versus ORIF versus closed reduction percutaneous fixation
	LCIII - LCII + SS & ST ligament torn and contralateral sacroiliac (SI) disruption	External fixation versus ORIF versus closed reduction percutaneous fixation
APC = Anterior posterior compression	Anterior posterior compression (APC) I - < 2 cm symphysis pubis, ± sacroiliac (SI) joint widening	Symptomatic treatment
	APCII-disrupted symphysis or anterior ring, SS & ST torn	Anterior external fixation versus ORIF versus closed reduction percutaneous fixation
	APCIII - APCII & post SI ligament (internal hemi-pelvectomy)	Same as APC II
VS = Vertical shear	Vertical Shear – APCIII & vertical displacement	Same as APC II
	CMI-Combination mechanism injury	Same as APC II

[53] Denis, F. The Three-Column Spine and its Significance in the Classification of Acute Thoracolumbar Spinal Injuries. Spine, 8:1983

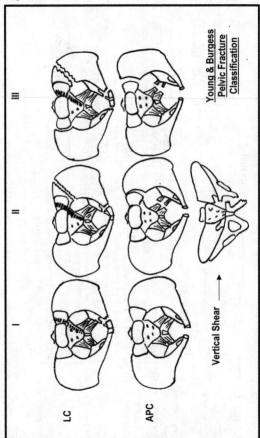

Young & Burgess
Pelvic Fracture
Classification

Vertical Shear ⟶

LC

APC

III

II

I

Pelvic Fractures with Hemodynamic Instability

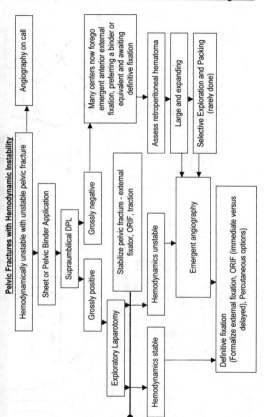

Hemodynamically unstable with unstable pelvic fracture

→ Angiography on call

Sheet or Pelvic Binder Application

Supraumbilical DPL

- Grossly negative → Many centers now forego emergent anterior external fixation, preferring a binder or equivalent and awaiting definitive fixation

  - Assess retroperitoneal hematoma
    - Large and expanding
    - Selective Exploration and Packing (rarely done)

- Grossly positive → Exploratory Laparotomy

Stabilize pelvic fracture - external fixator, ORIF, traction

- Hemodynamics unstable → Emergent angiography
- Hemodynamics stable → Definitive fixation (Formalize external fixation, ORIF (immediate versus delayed), Percutaneous options)

Pelvis Fractures

Injury/Eponym	Classification	Treatment
Acetabular Fracture (see page 145)	**Letournel**	Non-operative-
	5 Simple fracture patterns	Roof arc angle > 45° as measured off the AP, iliac oblique, and obturator oblique.
	Posterior wall	Relative non-operative indications-
	Posterior column	Secondary congruence of the acetabulum with a
	Anterior wall	associated both column fracture
	Anterior column	ORIF- unstable joint, incongruous joint
	Simple transverse	
	5 Complex/associated fracture patterns	
	T-shaped	
	Posterior wall and column	
	Transverse posterior wall	
	Anterior with posterior hemitransverse	
	Both columns	

Neck Shaft Angle
124° ± 7°

Head

Neck

Inter-
trochanteric

Sub-
Trochanteric

Hip Fractures

Simple Acetabular Fractures (5 types)

- Posterior Wall
- Posterior Column
- Anterior Wall
- Anterior Column
- Transverse

Letournel Classification of Acetabular Fractures

Complex/Associated Acetabular Fractures (5 types)

- T-Shaped
- Posterior Column & Posterior Wall
- Transverse & Posterior Wall
- Anterior with Posterior Hemitransverse
- Both Columns

Periprosthetic Femur Fracture Classification and Treatment

Type	Fracture Location	Recommended Treatment
I	Trochanteric region	Non operative
II	Proximal metaphysis/diaphysis not involving stem tip	Non operative or cerclage fixation
IIIA	Diaphyseal fracture at stem tip Disruption of prosthetic interface (< 5%)	Long-stem ingrowth revision or ORIF: plate with screws ± cerclage ORIF: cortical struts with cerclage cables
IIIB	Diaphyseal fracture at stem tip Disruption of prosthetic interface (> 25%)	Cemented stem: long-stem ingrowth revision Ingrowth stem: long-stem ingrowth revision or ORIF: plate with screws ± cerclage ORIF: cortical struts with cerclage cables
IIIC	Supracondylar fracture at tip of a long stem prosthesis	Non operative if stable or ORIF: plate with screws ± cerclage ORIF: custom intramedullary rod extension to prosthesis
IV	Supracondylar fracture distal to the stem tip	Non operative if stable or ORIF: plate with screws (must extend proximal to stem tip) ORIF: supracondylar intramedullary nail Long stem ingrowth revision

Adapted from Miller MD (ed.): Review of Orthopaedics, 3rd ed. Philadelphia, WB Saunders, 2000, page 252, with permission

Hip Fractures

Injury/Eponym	Classification	Treatment
Femoral Neck	**Garden** I - Incomplete, valgus impacted II - Complete, non-displaced III - Complete, partial displaced IV - Complete fracture and displacement	Closed reduction internal fixation (3 screws) versus Hip screw ± derotational screw Hemi arthroplasty-elderly, sick, pathologic fracture, rheumatoid arthritis, patient with a seizure disorder, Parkinson's disease, Garden types III & IV, total hip arthroplasty for patient with pre-existing osteoarthrosis

Hip Fractures (Continued)

Injury/Eponym	Classification	Treatment
Femoral Neck (Continued)	Blickenstaff/Morris (stress fractures)	
	I - Callus	Weight bearing - advanced weight bearing as tolerated
	II - Non-displaced	Tension side - closed reduction internal fixation Compression - like type I
	III - Displaced	Closed reduction internal fixation (acute), ORIF (subacute/chronic)
Intertrochanteric	Boyd/Griffin	Closed reduction internal fixation with sliding compression screw
	I - Non-displaced	Unstable = type III or postero-medial comminution
	II - Displaced	No sliding hip screw with type III (reverse obliquity)
	III - Reverse obliquity	Osteopenia/pathologic fracture - consider calcar replacing hemi arthroplasty
	IV - Subtrochanteric spike	
	Evans	
	Stable/Unstable	
Greater Trochanter	Non-displaced	Activity modification
	Displaced	> 1 cm ORIF
Lesser Trochanter	Non-displaced	Activity modification
	Displaced	> 2 cm ORIF
Sub-trochanteric	Seinsheimer	
	I - Non/minimally displaced	Intramedullary nail-locked
	II - 2-part	Intramedullary nail-locked
	III - 3-part	Reconstruction nail or condylar plate/screw
	IV - Comminuted	Reconstruction nail or condylar plate/screw
	V - Subtrochanteric-inter trochanteric	Sliding compression screw + long side plate (older), condylar blade (young)

Hip Dislocations

Injury/Eponym	Classification	Treatment

Anterior	Epstein
	I - Superior
	  A - No fracture
	  B - Head fracture
	  C - Acetabular fracture
	II - Inferior
	  A - No fracture
	  B - Head fracture
	  C - Acetabular fracture
		Emergent closed reduction, open if irreducible
		ORIF if irreducible unstable, or intra articular bodies
		Methods:
		Stimson - Prone, leg hanging off table, immobilize pelvis, knee/ankle at 90°, distal traction, & gentle rotation
		Allis - Supine, stabilize pelvis, lateral traction to inner thigh, long traction to femur, slight hip flexion, & rotation
		Reverse Bigelow - Supine, hip partial flexion & abduction, distal jerk, no reduction then add internal rotation and extend

Posterior	Thompson/ Epstein I - No/minimal fracture II - Posterior acetabular rim III - Comminuted rim IV - Acetabular floor V - Femoral Head	Emergent closed reduction, open if necessary ORIF if irreducible unstable, or intra articular bodies **Methods:** Stimson-Prone, leg hanging off table, immobilize pelvis, knee/hip at 90°, distal traction, & gentle rotation Allis-Supine, stabilize pelvis, traction inline with deformity, hip flexion to 90°, & rotation Bigelow-Supine, stabilize pelvis, hand holds ankle- forearm behind knee to apply long traction, hip flexed to 90°or more, abduction, external rotation, extension to lever head into acetabulum

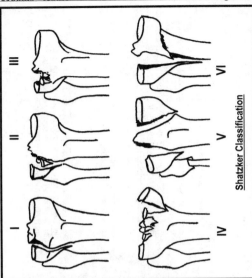

Shatzker Classification

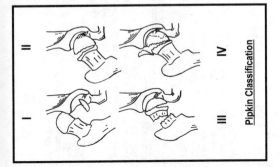

Pipkin Classification

Hip Dislocations

Injury/Eponym	Classification	Treatment
Posterior with Femoral head (Type V Thomas-Epstein)	Pipkin (see page 149)	All - Emergent closed reduction
	I - Head caudad	Excise loose fragment if blocks motion or displaced, ORIF if large fragment
	II - Head cephalad	ORIF if large fragment or part of weight bearing dome
	III - Femoral head & neck	ORIF (young), selective arthroplasty (older)
	IV - Associated acetabular fracture	ORIF (young), selective arthroplasty (older)

Femoral Shaft Fractures

Injury/Eponym	Classification	Treatment
Femur (2cm from Lesser trochanter to 8cm above joint)	Winquist I - Transverse, <25% butterfly II - Transverse, 25 - 50% butterfly III - > 50% butterfly, no comminution IV - comminuted, no cortical contact V - segmental.	Locked intramedullary nail (external fixator, ORIF, traction)
Femoral neck & shaft		Closed reduction percutaneous pinning versus ORIF of neck (first). Intramedullary rod or plate for shaft versus cephalomedullary nail
Femoral shaft/ tibial shaft	"Floating Knee"	Intramedullary rod femur and tibia, consider external fixator for tibia or femur (based on extent of soft tissue injury.

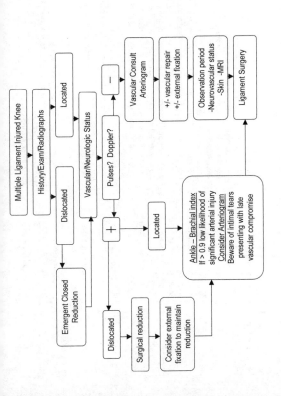

Multiple Ligament Injured Knee

History/Exam/Radiographs

Dislocated → Located

Emergent Closed Reduction

Vascular/Neurologic Status

Pulses? Doppler?

−

Vascular Consult
Arteriogram

+/- vascular repair
+/- external fixation

Observation period
-Neurovascular status
-Skin -MRI

Ligament Surgery

+

Located

Dislocated

Surgical reduction

Consider external fixation to maintain reduction

Ankle – Brachial index
If > 0.9 low likelihood of significant arterial injury
Consider Arteriogram
Beware of intimal tears presenting with late vascular compromise

Knee fractures

Injury/Eponym	Classification	Treatment
Supra-condylar	AO	> 6 - 8 cm proximal - intramedullary nail anterograde
		< 6 - 8 cm condylar blade plate/screw, retrograde nail, consider LISS (Synthes) versus traditional plating/internal fixation for displaced intra articular fractures
Patella	Non-displaced, transverse, lower pole, upper pole, comminuted, vertical	Non-displaced = cylinder cast
		ORIF (tension band) - no active extension, > 2mm separation, incongruent joint, consider excising comminuted fragment and reattaching tendon
Tibial Plateau (treatment based on joint stability, displacement and articular congruity)	Shatzker (see page 149) I - Split lateral plateau	Closed treatment if non-displaced, closed reduction percutaneous fixation if no incarcerated meniscus by scope or MRI, ORIF if incarcerated meniscus
	II - Split/depression lateral plateau	Closed treatment if non-displaced, ORIF with elevation of the depressed joint surface for > 3 mm displacement (some accept as much as 4 – 10 mm) or instability
	III - Isolated depression	Closed treatment, ORIF (similar criteria as type II)
	IV - Medial split/depression	Closed treatment (only for selected non-displaced), otherwise ORIF
	V - Bicondylar	ORIF versus external fixation
	VI - Type V & metaphyseal extension	ORIF versus external fixation
Tibial Spine	Meyer/Mckeever I-Anterior elevation	Long leg cast 15 - 20° of flexion x 4 - 6 weeks
	II-Anterior 1/3-1/2 elevated	Long leg cast 15 - 20° of flexion x 4 - 6 weeks, unstable = MRI & treat like III
	IIIA-Displaced	MRI, arthroscopic fixation
	IIIB- Displaced & rotated	MRI, arthroscopic fixation

Knee fractures (Continued)

Injury/Eponym	Classification	Treatment
Tibial Tubercle		ORIF

Knee Dislocation/Soft Tissue Injury

Quadriceps rupture		Surgical repair
Patellar tendon rupture		Surgical repair
Patellar Dislocation		Conservative treatment, Rule out osteochondral injury
		Evaluate Medial patello-femoral ligament, consider repair
Proximal Tibia-Fibula Dislocation	Ogden -Subluxation -Posteromedial -Anterolateral -Superior	Treat subluxation conservatively Dislocations – closed reduction (knee 90°) ± anesthesia, Limited immobilization
Knee Dislocation	Descriptive of tibia in relation to femur	See algorithm page 151

Tibia/Fibular Fractures

Tibia	Johner/Wruhs
	A-Simple 1 - Spiral
	           2 - Oblique
	           3 - Transverse
	B-Butterfly 1 - By torsion
	           2 - One (bend)
	           3 - Multiple (bend)
	C-Comminuted 1 - Torsion
	               2 - Segmental
	               3 - Crush
		Closed reduction & cast = low energy, minimal displaced, isolated
		All others – intramedullary nail, external fixator, plate
		
		**Maintain a high index of suspicion for compartment syndrome
		
		Acceptable reduction limits 5° varus & valgus, 10° anterior & posterior, 10° rotation, & 1 cm shortening (Rockwood & Green, Fractures in Adults, 4th ed. Lippincott-Raven, Baltimore 1996, p. 2139)

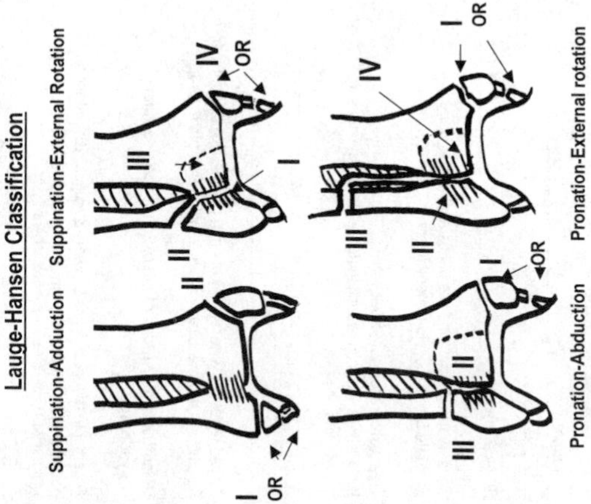

Lauge-Hansen Classification

Suppination-Adduction

Suppination-External Rotation

Pronation-External rotation

Pronation-Abduction

Weber Classification

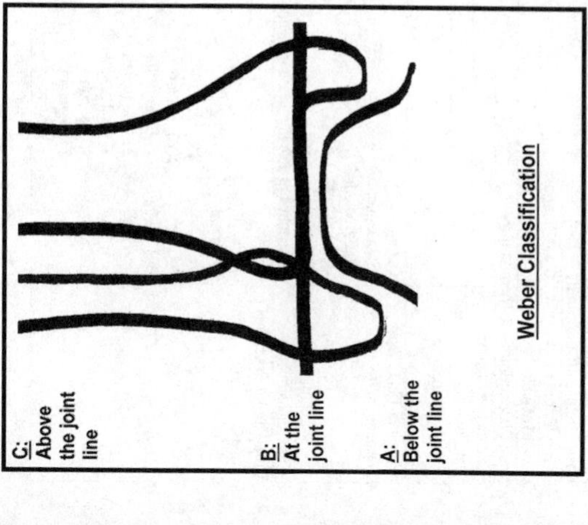

C:
Above
the joint
line

B:
At the joint line

A:
Below the
joint line

Ankle Fractures/Dislocations

Injury/Eponym	Classification	Treatment
Ankle Fractures	Lauge-Hansen	Bimalleolar fracture or equivalent ORIF
	Supination-Adduction	Selected non-operative treatment for non-displaced
AITFL = Anterior inferior talo-fibular ligament	1 - Lateral malleolus or lateral collateral ligament	fractures without syndesmotic injury
	2 - Medial malleolus – shear	Syndesmotic screw for widened mortise
PITFL= Posterior inferior talo-fibular ligament	Supination-External rotation	
	1 - AITFL	
	2 - Lateral malleolus (spiral)	
	3 - Posterior malleolus or PITFL	
	4 - Medial malleolus or deltoid ligament	
	Pronation-Abduction	
	1 - Medial malleolus or deltoid	
	2 - AITFL /PITFL or posterior malleolus	
	3 - Lateral malleolus	
	Pronation-External rotation	
	1 - Medial malleolus or deltoid	
	2 - AITFL or bony avulsion	
	3 - High fibular	
	4 - Posterior malleolus or PITFL	
	Danis/Weber	In general
	A - Fibular fracture below the syndesmosis	A = Closed
	B - At the syndesmosis	B & C = ORIF ± syndesmotic screw
	C - Above the syndesmosis	

Tibial/Fibular Fractures

Injury/Eponym	Classification	Treatment
Tibial Stress Fracture		Activity modification
Fibular Shaft		Cast for pain control
Tibial Plafond	Ruedi/Allgower	
	I - Minimally displaced	Non operative stable/non-displaced fractures
	II - Incongruous	II & III–ORIF versus external fixation if displaced (min. invasive)
	III - Comminuted	Soft tissues are the key. You can always bridge and wait
Achilles Tendon Rupture		Casting (higher rerupture) versus surgical repair (skin necrosis)

Foot Fractures and Dislocations

Injury/Eponym	Classification	Treatment
Stress fracture, *March*	2nd Metatarsal, Calcaneus	Activity modification and short leg cast
Posterior Talar Process *Shepard's*		Short leg cast or excision of fragments
Lateral Talar Process		Short leg cast, excision of fragments, or ORIF
Talar Head	Non-displaced	Non-operative
	Displaced	ORIF or fragment excision
Talar Body		ORIF
Talar Neck	Hawkins/Canale	
Aviators Astralgus	I - Non-displaced (< 1 mm), vertical	Short leg non-walking cast
	II - Displaced + subtalar subluxation dislocation	ORIF - anatomic reduction
	III - Displaced & talar body dislocation	ORIF - anatomic reduction
	IV - With talar head dislocation	ORIF - anatomic reduction

> **Hawkin's sign** –
> Relative osteoporosis of the talar dome at 6 - 8 weeks signifies an intact vascular supply (JBJS 52A:991-1002, 1970).

Foot Fractures and Dislocations (Continued)

Injury/Eponym	Classification	Treatment
Subtalar Dislocation *Basketball foot*	Calcaneus – medial	Closed reduction/cast, open reduction if irreducible
	Calcaneus - lateral	
Calcaneal Fractures	Extra-articular	Short leg non walking cast versus ORIF
	Anterior process	
	Tuberosity	
	Medial process	
	Sustentaculum	
	Body	
	Intra-articular (see page 158)	CT scan beneficial, selective ORIF for articular displacement and calcaneal body widening
		Restore congruous joint surface
Mid-Tarsal Injury	Medial stress	Closed reduction percutaneous fixation
	Longitudinal stress	
	Lateral stress	
	Plantar stress	
	Crush	
Navicular	Cortical avulsion	Reduce/pin large fragment
	Tuberosity fracture	ORIF (screw/washer)
	Body fracture	ORIF displaced
	Stress fracture	Short leg non walking cast
Cuboid, *Nutcracker*		ORIF & bone graft or external fixator (restore lateral column)
Tarso-metatarsal fracture/dislocation *Lis Franc*	Homolateral	Closed reduction percutaneous fixation versus
	Isolated	ORIF (usual – reliably reduces joints)
	Divergent	

CT Classification of Calcaneal Fractures
(Sander's Clin. Orthop. 290:87-95, 1993.)

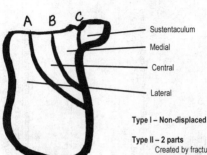

Sustentaculum

Medial

Central

Lateral

Type I – Non-displaced

Type II – 2 parts
Created by fracture line A, B, or C and a secondary fracture line in the axial plane from line A, B, or C laterally to the lateral cortex.

Type III – 3 parts
Fractures lines A & B, B & C, or A & C creating 3 parts

Type IV – Comminuted
Fracture lines A, B, & C

The primary fracture line
Defined as a line that travels from the plantar aspect dorsalward to the posterior facet of the subtalar joint when observed from the side. In the axial plane the line travels obliquely plantarmedial to dorsolateral.

2 Main fracture fragments
anteromedial
posterolateral

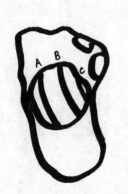

Foot Fractures and Dislocations (Continued) Page 157

Injury/Eponym	Classification	Treatment
Metatarsal	Shaft	Closed reduction/selective fixation
	Head	Closed reduction ± cast/pinning
(Pseudo-Jones zones I & II)	5th metatarsal	
	Zone I	Short leg walking cast
	Zone II	Short leg cast ± weight bearing
True Jones (zone III)	Zone III	Short leg non weight bearing cast x 6 weeks, ORIF (late or athlete)
Metatarsophalangeal Joint Dislocation		Reduce/buddy tape ± pinning (unstable)
Phalanges		Buddy tape ± cast or cast shoe
		Selective ORIF versus percutaneous pinning intra-articular displaced fracture

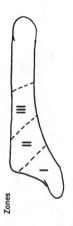

Zones

5th Metatarsal Fracture

Pediatric Trauma - Wrist and Hand Fractures

Injury/Eponym	Classification	Treatment
Distal phalanx fractures	Extra-physeal A - Transverse B - Longitudinal split C - Comminuted	Closed reduction/splinting-stable Pinning-unstable
Seymour fracture		
Distal phalanx fracture with a nail bed injury (any distal phalanx physeal)	Physeal (Mallet finger) A - Salter-Harris I or II B - Salter-Harris III or IV C - A & dislocation D - Avulsed extensor & Salter-Harris fracture	Extension splinting x 6 weeks (rarely operative) Type B with large dorsal fragment > 50% or significant volar sag may need operative intervention Type C & D need operative intervention to restore joint surface and extensor continuity
Jersey or reverse mallet (phalanx E)	E-Volar	Type E requires tendon repair, retraction proximal to the A4 pulley likely means disruption of the vincular system – repair acutely (< 1 week)
Proximal & middle phalanx	A - Physeal -extra-articular Salter-Harris II -intra-articular III/IV	Closed reduction/splint, percutaneous pinning if unstable, ORIF joint incongruity (> 25% of joint surface, displacement > 1.5 mm)
	B – Shaft	Closed reduction ± percutaneous pinning (angulation > 20° age < 10 years, 10 - 15° age > 10 years), ORIF if needed
	C - Phalangeal neck	Closed reduction/splint, percutaneous pinning (often), ORIF if needed
	D - Articular/condylar	ORIF (usually necessary) if displaced or incongruous
	Jammed finger	Buddy tape
Proximal interphalangeal joint dislocation (PIPJ)	Dislocation	Reduction under local anesthesia. Without collateral or volar plate instability – buddy tape x 3 weeks. Collateral instability – immobilize @ 20 – 30° flexion x 3 weeks, then buddy tape. Volar plate laxity – dorsal splint at 45° or extension block splinting x 3 weeks

Wrist and Hand Fractures (Continued)

Injury/Eponym	Classification	Treatment
PIPJ (continued)	Open injuries	Irrigation and debridement, reduction then treat as closed
Metacarpal fractures	A - Epiphyseal and physeal	Closed, unstable = percutaneous pinning, displaced head splitting need ORIF
	B - Neck fracture	Closed, unstable = percutaneous pinning
	C - Shaft fracture	Closed, unstable = percutaneous pinning, ORIF rare
	D - Metacarpal base fracture	Closed reduction percutaneous pinning, ORIF if irreducible
Finger metacarpal dislocation	Dorsal (index finger most common)	Closed reduction usually unsuccessful, Operative reduction as needed
Thumb metacarpal dislocation	Farabeuf Incomplete dislocation	All – closed reduction versus open reduction for failed closed, cast x 3 weeks (Collaterals intact)
	Complete simple	(Collaterals torn & volar plate torn and not in joint)
	Complete complex	(Collaterals torn & volar plate torn and interposed in joint)
Thumb metacarpal fractures	Head	Closed reduction (treat like finger metacarpal fractures)
	Shaft	Accept angulation < 20° (treat like finger metacarpal fractures)
	Metacarpal base	Closed reduction, ± percutaneous pinning for instability
	A -Distal to physis	Displaced type D fracture = ORIF, external fixation (severe open fractures), traction (complex injuries)
	B - Salter-Harris II, fragment ulnar	
	C - Salter-Harris II, fragment radial	Displaced Salter-Harris fractures need ORIF
	D - Salter-Harris III or IV	
CMCJ dislocation	Extremely rare	Closed reduction percutaneous pinning
Scaphoid	A-Distal Pole	Cast immobilization (long arm thumb spica cast)
	1-Extra articular, 2-Intra-articular	Significantly displaced (considered on skeletal age and angulation
	B-Mid waist	>10° and > 1 mm displacement) or additional carpal injury consider
	C-Proximal pole	open reduction percutaneous pinning versus internal fixation

Radius/Ulnar Shaft (Fracture/Dislocation)

Injury/Eponym	Classification	Treatment
Distal radius	Salter-Harris classification	Closed reduction/Cast
		Operative indications: soft tissue injury, associated proximal ipsilateral fracture, failed closed reduction, open, comminuted intra-physeal, carpal tunnel symptoms, compartment syndrome
Distal ulna	A - Transphyseal	Closed reduction/cast
	B - Intraphyseal (styloid)	Open reduction for failed Closed reduction
Radius and ulna *Both bone* Acceptable angulation see chart below	Greenstick Compression Complete	Majority Closed reduction /cast
		Closed reduction percutaneous pinning indications: severe swelling, ipsilateral fracture, re reduction (External fixation, open reduction uncommon)
		Limits of Acceptable Alignment - (Rockwood CA, Wilkins KE, Beaty JH. Fractures In Children, 4th ed. Lippincott-Williams & Wilkins, 1997, page 524 & Green NE, Swiontkowski MF Skeletal Trauma in Children: Vol 3. W.B. Saunders, Phila, 1998, page 203)
		< 8 years:
		15° angulation, 45° malrotation, 100% displacement, complete loss of radial bow
		♂ 9 - 14 years or ♀: 9 - 16 years;
		10° angulation, 30° malrotation, 100% displacement, partial loss of radial bow

Acceptable Angulation Distal Metaphysis (Volar-Dorsal Plane) - 30° with 5 yr growth remaining, subtract 5° for each year less
Acceptable Angulation Distal Metaphyseal (Radial-Ulnar Plane) - 20° with 5 yr growth remaining
Reduction goals - 80% apposition, 100% correction

Radius/Ulnar Shaft (Fracture/Dislocation)

Injury/Eponym	Classification	Treatment
Ulnar fracture/radial head dislocation	**Bado**	
	I - Anterior dislocation of the radial head with a fracture of the ulnar diaphysis	Reduce (traction/flexion), long arm cast - flexion/supination [most common ~ 70%]
Monteggia	II - Posterior dislocation of the radial head with an ulnar diaphyseal or metaphyseal fracture with posterior angulation	Reduce (traction/extension), long arm cast some extension
	III - Lateral or anterolateral dislocation of the radial head with a fracture of the ulnar metaphysis	Reduce (extension/pressure), long arm cast 90° flexion /supination
	IV - Anterior dislocation of the radial head, fracture of the middle 1/3 of the radius, and an ulna fracture at the same or more proximal level	Reduce (supination), ± ORIF
Radial Head Subluxation	*Nursemaid's* (see page 167)	Flexion, supination, pressure over radial head
Radial head dislocation		Reduce (supination/pressure), long arm cast 100° flexion, supination
Ulnar fracture/ radial neck fracture	Minimally displaced head	Reduce ± ORIF
	Displaced head	
Radius fracture/ distal radioulnar joint dislocation	*Galeazzi*	Reduce (traction/supination), long arm cast 90° flexion/supination Closed reduction percutaneous pinning if reduction unstable > 12 year old & failed closed reduction = ORIF

Elbow

Injury/Eponym	Classification	Treatment
Supracondylar	I - Non-displaced	Long arm cast - 90° Flexion, forearm neutral
Extension	II - Displaced, posterior cortex intact	Closed reduction, long arm cast > 90° versus percutaneous pinning
	III - No cortical contact (posterior medial & posterior lateral)	Closed reduction percutaneous pinning
Supracondylar	I - Non-displaced	Long arm cast versus posterior splint
Flexion	II - Displaced & contact	Closed reduction, Long arm cast versus percutaneous pinning
	III - No contact	Closed versus open Reduction percutaneous pinning
		Be careful of neurovascular status with flexion > 90°
Distal humeral physeal separation	DeLee	
	A - < 12 mo, Salter-Harris I	Closed reduction & cast
	B - 1 yr - 3 yr, Salter-Harris I	Closed reduction percutaneous pinning
	C - 3 - 12 yr, Salter-Harris II	Closed reduction percutaneous pinning
Lateral condyle fractures	Milch	
	I - Salter-Harris IV, fracture thru capitello-trochlear groove	< 2 mm displaced - closed reduction/cast and close F/U
		> 2 mm - closed reduction percutaneous pinning
	II - Salter-Harris II, fracture thru trochlea	Grossly unstable = open reduction percutaneous pinning
Capitellum fracture	Hahn-Steinthal (see page 133)	Closed reduction/cast versus ORIF
	Kocher-Lorenz	Excise versus ORIF
Medial condyle fracture	Kilfoyle	
	I - Fracture to physis	Splint versus cast
	II - Complete, non displaced	Closed reduction/cast versus percutaneous pinning
	III - Displaced	Closed or open reduction/percutaneous pinning v. internal fixation

Elbow (Continued)

Injury/Eponym	Classification	Treatment
Medial epicondylar apophysis	Acute Injuries Non/minimally displaced Displaced Incarcerated (without dislocation) (with dislocation)	Non-operative = non/minimally displaced, displaced low demand Operative indications (absolute) = irreducible incarcerated Operative indications (relative) = ulnar nerve dysfunction, high demand function
Little Leaguer elbow	Chronic tension	
T-Condylar	Toniolo/Wilkins I – Non-displaced	Closed reduction percutaneous pinning versus traction
	II – Displaced, no metaphyseal comminution	ORIF
	III – Metaphyseal comminution	Limited open reduction and traction
Elbow dislocation	Proximal radio-ulnar joint intact A - Posterior (posterior-medial & Posterior-lateral) B - Anterior C - Medial D - Lateral Proximal radio-ulnar joint dislocation A - Divergent (anterior-posterior & medial-lateral) B - Radio-ulnar translocation	Young = Sedation, closed reduction Older > 9 years old = general anesthesia, closed reduction Aftercare = Active elbow flexion at 5 days, sling at 10 days

Elbow (Continued)

Injury/Eponym	Classification	Treatment
Lateral epicondylar apophysis		Immobilization, incarceration operative intervention
Olecranon apophysis	I - Apophysitis II - Incomplete stress III - Complete fracture A - Pure apophyseal B-Apophysis & metaphysis	Non-displaced = splint/cast in extension Displaced = ORIF versus percutaneous pinning
Olecranon metaphysis	A - Flexion B - Extension (1-Valgus, 2-Varus) C - Shear	Non-displaced = cast in extension Significantly displaced = ORIF
Radial head & neck	Group I - Head 1 - Valgus fracture A - Salter-Harris I/II B - Salter-Harris IV C - Metaphyseal fracture 2 - With elbow dislocation D - Reduction injury E - Dislocation injury Group II - Neck 1 - Angular 2 - Torsional Group III-Stress 1 - Osteochondritis Dessicans 2 - Physeal injury + neck angulation	< 30°, no angulation = long arm cast versus posterior splint, and early range of motion > 30° = closed reduction (general anesthesia) using flexion-pronation, long arm cast x 10-14days > 45° = closed reduction (general anesthesia) using flexion-pronation, ace wrap, or percutaneous pins, then long arm cast x 10-14days Fixed 40° angulation, < 60° pronation/supination, 3 mm translation, head completely displaced = wire reduction, open reduction ± internal fixation

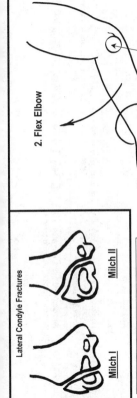

2. Flex Elbow

1. Supinate Forearm

Gentle Pressure over Radial head

Lateral Condyle Fractures

Milch I

Milch II

Nursemaid's Elbow
- Refusal to move arm
- Pain at elbow
- May give characteristic history

Treatment
- Supinate forearm
- Flex elbow with thumb on radial head
- Radial head should relocate
- Success is walking away to return later and see the child using the arm

Shoulder

Injury/Eponym	Classification	Treatment
Humeral shaft	Birth injury	Splint
	0 - 3 years	Collar & cuff
	3 - 12 years	Velpeau
	> 12 years	Sugar tong splint
Proximal humerus	Salter-Harris Neer-Horowitz	Minimally displaced = splint
	I - ≤ 5mm displaced	Unstable ± percutaneous pinning
	II - ≤ 1/3 shaft	Soft tissue interposition or open fracture - ORIF
	III - ≤ 2/3 shaft	2 studies support non-operative treatment even in the face
	IV - Complete shaft	of severe displacement or angulation (Baxter et al JBJS(Br)86;68:570-73 & Beringer et al JPO 98;18:31-37)
Midshaft clavicle	0 - 2 years old	Supportive
	> 2 years old	Figure-of-8, sling
Medial clavicle	Salter-Harris I & II	Sling
Sternoclavicular joint	Anterior	Sling
	Posterior	Closed versus Open reduction
Medial clavicular physis is the last to close (~ 25 yo), sternoclavicular dislocations usually represent Salter-Harris type II fractures		
Glenohumeral dislocation	Traumatic	Closed reduction, Rehabilitation, ± reconstruction/repair
	Anterior & Posterior	
Scapular fracture	Anatomic	Similar to adults
Lateral clavicle	I - Non-displaced, intact ligaments	Sling, figure-of-8, consider ORIF for certain type II's
	IIA - Fracture medial to Coraco-clavicular ligaments	
	IIB - Conoid ligament tear	
	III - Fracture into acromioclavicular joint	

Shoulder (Cont.)

Injury/Eponym	Classification	Treatment
Acromioclavicular joint	I - Sprain	I - III = Closed treatment
	II - Partial tear dorsal periosteum	
	III - Large tear dorsal periosteum	
	IV - Posterior displacement	Closed reduction versus open reduction/repair
	V - Significant superior displaced	Open reduction, repair, reconstruction
	VI -Inferior displaced	Closed reduction versus open reduction
Scapulo - Thoracic dissociation		ABC's, reconstruction/repair

Spine Fractures

Injury/Eponym	Classification	Treatment
SCIWORA	Spinal Cord Injury Without Radiographic Abnormality	High index of suspicion, CT versus MRI
Occiput - C1 dislocation	High mortality	Occiput - C3 fusion
C1 - Atlas fracture		Minerva versus HALO vest
C1 - C2 injuries	Ligament disruption	C1-C2 fusion
	Rotatory subluxation	
	I - No anterior shift	< 1 week - soft collar, NSAIDS
	II - Anterior < 5mm	< 1 month - relax, traction, bedrest
	III - Anterior > 5mm	1 – 3 month - HALO
	IV - Posterior shift	> 3 month - C1-2 fusion
C2 fracture *Hangman's*		Minerva cast versus HALO immobilization

Spine (Continued)

Injury/Eponym	Classification	Treatment
C2 - C7 fracture	Posterior ligament injuries	Usually non-operative
	Wedge/compression fracture	Unstable = fuse
	Distraction/shear fracture	
	Fracture-dislocation	
	Facet dislocation/listhesis	
Thoracic & lumbar fractures	Flexion	Usually non-operative
	With compression	Operative fixation - unstable, open wound, progressive neurological deficit, slipped vertebral apophysis
	Without compression	
	Distraction	
	Shear	

Hip Fracture & Dislocations

Injury/Eponym	Classification	Treatment
Hip fracture	Delbet	
	I - Transepiphyseal (with & without dislocation)	Closed reduction & spica cast versus open reduction percutaneous pinning (open treatment more common with head dislocation)
	II - Transcervical (45 – 50%)	Closed reduction versus open reduction percutaneous pinning (AVN increases with displacement)
	III - Cervico-trochanteric	
	Displaced	Closed reduction versus open reduction percutaneous pinning/compression screw
	Non displaced	Abduction spica cast, close F/U, ORIF indicated for displacement in cast
	IV - Intertrochanteric	Traction then casting versus closed reduction & compression screw
Stress fracture	Devas Tension	Percutaneous pinning
	Compression	Non weight bearing
Hip dislocation	Anterior	Closed reduction, open reduction (irreducible), CT scan (Intra articular bodies)
	Posterior	

Pelvic & Acetabulum Fractures (Continued)

Injury/Eponym	Classification	Treatment
Pelvic fracture	**Key & Conwell**	**Restore joint congruity and hip stability**
	I - No ring break	
	A - Avulsion fracture (ASIS, AIIS, Ischial tuberosity)	Short period of rest, relax muscles associated with spine/ tuberosity, advance partial weight bearing as tolerated
	B - Pubis/ischium	Short bedrest, advance partial weight bearing as tolerated
	C - Iliac wing	Short bedrest, advance partial weight bearing as tolerated
	D - Sacrum/coccyx	Short bedrest, advance partial weight bearing as tolerated
	II - Single break	
Duverney →	A - 2 ipsilateral rami	Short bedrest, advance partial weight bearing as tolerated
	B - Fracture/subluxation symphysis	Short bedrest, advance weight bearing as tolerated
	C - Fracture/subluxation sacroiliac joint	Short bedrest, advance weight bearing as tolerated
	III - Double break	
	A - 2 anterior fracture/dislocation	Bedrest x 6 wk, advance partial weight bearing as tolerated
Straddle →	B - 2 vertical fracture/dislocation	Bedrest x 6 wk, advance partial weight bearing as tolerated
Malgaigne →	C - Severe multiple fractures	Bedrest, traction, ORIF > 3 cm
	IV - Acetabular fracture	
	A - Small fragment, + dislocation	Treat as pelvic fracture
	B - Linear, non-displaced pelvic fracture	Restore congruity
	C - Linear, unstable joint	ORIF
	D - Due to central fracture/dislocation	ORIF

Femoral Shaft Fractures

Injury/Eponym	Classification	Treatment

Femur fracture	Anatomic/ descriptive
	
	Treatment is very variable between centers!
		0 – 6 mo
		  Stable - Pavlik
		  Unstable - immediate spica or traction & delayed spica
		6 mo - 5 yr
		  < 3 cm shortening - immediate spica
		  > 3 cm initial, > 2 cm in spica traction - delayed spica
		  Polytrauma - external fixator, flexible intramedullary nails
		6 - 11yr
		  Stable - immediate spica
		  Unstable - traction, delayed spica, external fixator,
		    flexible intramedullary nail
		12 - adult
		  Flexible/rigid intramedullary nail based on maturity & fracture
		    Configuration
		Limits of Acceptable Angulation – (Rockwood CA, Wilkins KE, Beaty JH. Fractures in Children, 4th ed. Lippincott-Williams & Wilkins, 1997, page 1201)
		0 – 2 years: 30° varus/valgus, 30° anterior/posterior, 15 mm short
		2 – 5 years: 15° varus/valgus, 20° anterior/posterior, 20 mm short
		6 – 10 years: 10° varus/valgus, 15° anterior/posterior, 15 mm short
		> 11 years: 5° varus/valgus, 10° anterior/posterior, 10 mm short

Subtrochanteric/ Supracondylar	Subtrochanteric Supracondylar	Traction & cast versus cast brace Stable - cast Unstable - closed versus open reduction internal fixation/percutaneous pinning

Knee Fractures & Dislocations

Injury/Eponym	Classification	Treatment
Floating knee	Letts/Vincent A - Diaphyseal/closed B - Metaphyseal/diaphyseal closed C - Epiphyseal/diaphyseal closed D - 1 fracture open E - both open	Fix 1, usually the tibia Fix femur if: Severe head trauma with posturing, skeletal maturity, severe soft tissue injury, irreducible closed
Distal femoral physeal fracture	Salter-Harris	I,II - Closed reduction, long leg cast III,IV - Closed reduction percutaneous pinning
Proximal tibial physeal fracture	Salter-Harris	Non displaced - long leg cast, 30° flexion Displaced - closed reduction percutaneous pinning
Tibial tubercle avulsion	Ogden I - Distal, secondary ossification center II - Junction 1 & 2 ossification centers III - Into knee joint	Non displaced, minimally displaced with active extension 0° - long leg cast Displaced - ORIF
Intercondylar eminence fracture	I - Incomplete, non displaced II - Hinged (posterior) III - Supinated/rotated	Attempt closed reduction, long leg cast in extension (neutral - 10°) ORIF if irreducible
Osteochondral fractures (knee)	33% bilateral, ♀ < ♂, 5 – 15 yr.	Initially treat with ↓ activity ± immobilization unless unstable or detached Operative treatment for failure on non-operative × 3 – 6 mo (arthroscopy) < 1 cm excise & drill; ≥ 1 cm consider open curettage, reduction, & fixation

Knee Fractures & Dislocations (Continued)

Injury/Eponym	Classification	Treatment
Patella fracture	Non displaced	Long leg cast
	Displaced (3 mm step off or 3 mm displaced)	ORIF (tension band)
	Periosteal sleeve (usually 8 - 12 yr)	ORIF ± tension band
Knee dislocation	Anatomic	Similar to adults except kids may be primarily repaired, isolated ligament injuries may be treated non-operatively
Patellar dislocation		Closed reduction, cylinder cast
		Intra articular osteochondral fracture may need excision versus ORIF
Tibio-fibular joint dislocation	Subluxation	Closed reduction, rest versus cast
	Anterior/lateral	
	Posterior/medial	
	Superior	

Tibia & Fibula Fracture

Tibia & fibular fracture	I - Proximal tibial metaphyseal fracture	Non displaced - long leg cast 10° flexion; Displaced - closed versus open reduction, long leg cast
	II - Distal tibial metaphyseal fracture	Non displaced - long leg cast; Displaced-closed reduction, long leg cast
***GOAL	III - Diaphyseal fracture	Non displaced - long leg cast; Displaced- closed versus open reduction, long leg cast, internal or external fixation
-<1cm short	Isolated tibial, isolated fibular, both	
-<10 °angulation	IV - Special	
	Toddler's	Long leg cast
	Bicycle spoke	Soft tissue reconstruction/stabilization
	Pathologic	Based on pathologic condition & fracture
		** Be sure to counsel for overgrowth and correction based on age

Ankle Fracture

Injury/Eponym	Classification	Treatment
Ankle fracture	**Supination-Inversion**	Closed versus open reduction, Cast ± percutaneous pinning or screw fixation
	-Transverse fibula, shear medial malleolus	
	Pronation/Eversion External rotation	**Restore ankle mortise/joint surface
	-High fibula, medial malleolar transverse physeal	
	Supination-Plantar flexion	
	-Transphyseal posterior	
	Supination-External rotation	
	-Oblique fibular, oblique tibial	
	Axial compression (Salter-Harris V)	
	<u>Juvenile Tillaux</u> (Salter-Harris III lateral tibial physis)	Tri-plane & Tillaux - Based on CT scan > 2 mm displacement & > 2 mm stepoff - ORIF, otherwise treat in long leg cast
	<u>Triplane</u> (Salter-Harris III tibia anterior lateral, Salter-Harris IV posterior medial)	

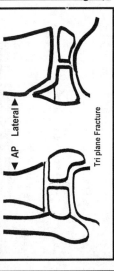

▲ AP   Lateral ▶

Tri plane Fracture

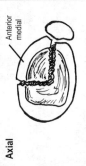

Axial

Anterior
medial

Juvenile Tillaux

Foot Fractures

Injury/Eponym	Classification	Treatment
Talus fracture	Neck	
	I - Non displaced	Cast
	II - Minimally displaced	Cast versus closed reduction percutaneous pinning
	III - Displaced	Closed reduction percutaneous pinning
Osteochondral fracture	Berndt/Harty	
	I - Subchondral trabecular injury	6 wk non weight bearing
	II - Incomplete separation	6 wk non weight bearing
	III - Complete, Non displaced	Arthroscopy- excision, microfracture, bone graft
	IV - Displaced	Arthroscopy- excision, microfracture, bone graft
Lesser tarsal fracture	Anatomic	Non-operative
Tarsometatarsal injuries	Hardcastle	
	A - Complete incongruity	Non displaced - cast
	B - Partial instability	Displaced - closed reduction percutaneous pinning versus open reduction percutaneous pinning versus internal fixation
	C - Divergent or total instability	
Metatarsals		Non-operative
		Unstable - closed reduction percutaneous pinning
Base 5th metatarsal	Jones	Short leg non walking cast, ORIF ± graft
	Pseudo-Jones	Short leg cast versus post operative shoe
Stress fracture		Activity modification
Phalangeal fracture		Non-operative

Foot Fractures (Continued)

Injury/Eponym	Classification	Treatment
Calcaneus	**Essex-Lopresti**	
	Type 1	Almost universally treated non-operatively
	A - Tuberosity/ apophysis	
	B - Sustentaculum tali	Older age and joint incongruity may need closed reduction percutaneous pinning versus ORIF
	C - Anterior process	
	D - Anterior inferior lateral process	
	E - Body avulsion	
	Type 2	
	Tuberosity posteriorly ± superior involvement	
	Type 3	
	Body, no subtalar involvement	
	Type 4	
	Subtalar involvement,	
	Non displaced	
	Type 5	
	Subtalar involvement, displaced	
	A - Tongue	
	B - Joint depression	
	Type 6	
	Non-classifiable	

Gustillo Classification[54]

Grade	Description	Antibiotic Choice[55]
I	Wound usually < 1cm, clean, minimal muscle contusion, low energy fracture (usually inside - out type wound)	1st generation cephalosporin such as cefazolin (Ancef) 1 gm IV q8h for 3 days (post wound closure)
II	Wound usually > 1 cm, significant soft tissue injury (flaps, avulsed skin, extensive muscle contusions, nerve injury), minimal to moderate crush component, moderate energy fractures, minimal comminution	1st generation cephalosporin such as cefazolin (Ancef) 1 gm IV q8h for 3 days (post wound closure)
III*	Wound usually > 10 cm, extensive soft tissue damage, high energy fractures, crush/shear injuries	cefazolin for 5 days plus gentamicin 2mg/kg and adjusted for serum levels or tobramycin, add 4 million units IV PCN G q6 hours for farmyard, highly contaminated, vascular injuries, or extensive crush injuries
IIIA	Soft tissue adequate for local coverage, segmental fracture, gunshot wound (GSW)	
IIIB	Periosteal stripping, exposed bone, extensive soft tissue injury, contamination, requires soft-tissue reconstructive surgery	Consider antibiotic bead pouch**
IIIC	Type III with vascular injury requiring repair	Consider antibiotic bead pouch**

*Automatic type III's – segmental fractures, farmyard injuries, fractures occurring in highly contaminated environments, shotgun wounds, high velocity gunshot wounds

**Antibiotic beads – tobramycin, gentamicin, vancomycin, or cephalosporin (0.5 – 1 g per 40 g cement)

Topical antibiotics in the irrigant are controversial but favored by some. Consider culture.[56]
Thorough debridement and irrigation is imperative in the treatment of all open injuries

---

[54] Gustillo RB, et. al. J Trauma 24:742-746, 1984

[55] Chapman MW and Olsen SA. Open Fractures in Rockwood and Green's Fractures in Adults. Philadelphia, Lippincott-Raven, 1996. pp 305-352

[56] Chapman, MW.: The Role of Intramedullary Fixation in Open Fractures, Clin Orthop., 212:27, 1986.

Open Hand injuries[57]

1. The patient as person and body
2. Other injuries; resuscitation
3. History
4. Physical Exam
5. Restoration of Blood Flow
6. Debridement (Repeat debridement)
7. Skeletal Stability
8. Repair of damaged structures
9. Appropriate timing of closure and coverage (When in doubt don't close)
10. Proper dressings and elevation
11. Tetanus prophylaxis and antibiotics (Antibiotics as useful "adjuncts". Antibiotics never substitute for adequate debridement. Cover severe wounds with oxacillin, or 1st generation cephalosporin)
12. Secondary reconstruction
13. Rehabilitation (As early as possible)
14. Tetanus prophylaxis

Mangled Extremity Severity Scale[58]

Component	Points
A. Skeletal and soft tissue injury	
Low energy (stab, simple fracture, low velocity (civilian) GSW)	1
Medium energy (open fracture, multiple fracture)	2
High energy (close range shotgun blast, high velocity GSW (military or assault weapon), crush injury)	3
Very high energy (same as high energy but add grossly contaminated or devitalized tissue)	4
B. Limb ischemia (double score time > 6 hr)	
Pulse decreased or gone with normal perfusion	1
Pulseless, paraesthetic, decreased capillary refill	2
Cool, paralyzed, insensate, anesthetic	3
C. Shock	
Transient hypotension (systolic < 90)	1
Persistent hypotension (systolic < 90)	2
D. Age (yeard)	
30 - 50	1
> 50	2

MSS score > 7 predicts the need for initial or eventual amputation, < 6 predicts a viable limb

---

[57] Brown PW. Open Injuries of the Hand In Green's Operative Hand Surgery, Philadelphia, Churchill Livingstone. 1607-1630

[58]Johansen, K. et. al.: J Trauma 30:568-573, 1990.

Red Cross Classification of War Wounds[59]

E – Entry
The maximum dimensions of the entry wound in cm.

X – Exit
The maximum dimension of the exit wound measured in cm. No exit = 0. When it isn't known which of the connecting wounds is entry or exit a "?" is placed between the scores.

C – Cavity
The wound is deemed to have a cavity if 2 fingers can be put into the wound before wound excision. This should not be confused with the phenomenon of temporary cavitation. This may be obvious before operation or assessed only after skin incision. C0 = no cavity, C1 = cavity.

F – Fracture
This can be assessed clinically or radiographically. F0 = no fracture. F1 = simple fracture, hole, or minimal comminution. F2 = clinically significant comminution.

V – Vital Structure Injured
V0 = non-vital injury. V1 = a wound involving viscera, major blood vessel (proximal to and including popliteal and brachial vessels), or the CNS

M – Metallic bodies (bullet or fragment visible radiographically)
M0 = none. M1 = one. M2 = Multiple.

*Use dashes when wound defies scoring in a category.

Abbreviated Injury Scale (AIS)/Injury Severity Score (ISS)

The AIS rates and compares injuries. Injuries are cataloged to nine body sections and assigned a numeric value (1 - 6) to each injury based on severity. The ISS summarizes the AIS data. It is the sum of the squares of the scores from the three most severely injured body regions. The six body regions used in the ISS are head/neck, face, chest, abdominal or pelvic contents, extremities or pelvic girdle, and external. ISS scores range from 1 - 75. A score of 6 in any region makes the ISS 75, regardless of other involved areas. ISS ≥ 18 defines a multiple trauma patient. ISS < 30 usually indicates a favorable prognosis, whereas > 60 is usually fatal.

[59] Coupland, RF. The Red Cross Classification of War Wounds: The E.X.C.F.V.M. Scoring System. World J Surg. 16: 910-917, 92. pp. 910-917.

Tumor/Orthopaedic Pathology

Age distribution of Various Common Bone Lesions

Age	Malignant	Benign
Birth to 5 yr.	Leukemia	Osteomyelitis
	Metastatic neuroblastoma	Osteofibrous dysplasia
	Metastatic rhabdomyosarcoma	Osteochondroma
		Chondroblastoma
10 - 25 years	Osteosarcoma	Eosinophilic granuloma
	Ewing's Sarcoma	Osteomyelitis
	Leukemia	Enchondroma
	Adamantinoma	Fibrous dysplasia
		Aneurysmal bone cyst
		Giant cell tumor
		Simple bone cyst
40 - 80 years	Metastatic bone disease	Hyperparathyroidism
	Myeloma	Paget's disease
	Lymphoma	Mastocytosis
	Paget's Sarcoma	
	Post-radiation Sarcoma	
	Malignant Fibrous Histiocytoma	

Staging System for Musculoskeletal Lesions (Enneking)

Stage	GTM	Description
IA	$G_1T_1M_0$	Low grade, intracompartmental, no metastasis
IB	$G_1T_2M_0$	Low grade, extracompartmental, no metastasis
IIA	$G_2T_1M_0$	High grade, intracompartmental, no metastasis
IIB	$G_2T_2M_0$	High grade extracompartmental, no metastasis
IIIA	$G_{1/2}T_1M_1$	Any grade, intracompartmental, metastasis
IIIB	$G_{1/2}T_2M_1$	Any grade, extracompartmental, metastasis

Grade: G1=low grade, less common, metastasis <25%, G2 = high grade, metastasis >25%
Tumor site: T1 intracompartmental, T2 extracompartmental. Metastasis: M0 no metastasis, M1 metastasis

General Guidelines for Prophylactic Fixation

Pattern of Bone Destruction	Purely lytic – high risk
	Purely blastic – low risk
Size	< 25% - 35% cortical destruction – low risk
	> 50% - 75% cortical destruction – high risk
Location	High risk regions – femur neck, subtrochanteric, diaphysis
Pain	Risk increased with activity related pain
Post irradiation	Fixation to improve pain and increase mechanical strength
Prognosis	Survival < 4 weeks – Non operative treatment

Adapted with permission from Frassica FJ, et. al. Metastatic Bone Disease. Instructional Course Lectures 49:458, 2000.

Scoring system to predict pathological fracture

Parameter	Score		
	1	2	3
Pain	None	Moderate	Activity related
Location	Upper extremity	Lower extremity	Peritrochanteric
Bone destruction	Blastic	Mixed	Lytic
Size	< 1/3	1/3 - 2/3	> 2/3
Fracture group: median 10, range 7 - 12, Non fracture group: median 7, range 4 - 9 Scores 9 or higher fixation recommended			

Reproduced from Mirels H: Metastatic disease in long bones: A proposed scoring system for diagnosing impending pathologic fractures. Clin Orthop 1989;249:256-264.

Skeletal fixation of metastatic carcinoma
- Goal is maximize function and minimize pain
- The goal is not to affect a cure in metastatic disease
- Skeletal fixation or radiation therapy can meet goals

Laboratory Studies in Evaluation of a New Tumor Patient

5 - 40 years	40 - 80 years
Complete blood count with differential	Complete blood count with differential
Peripheral blood smear	Erythrocyte sedimentation rate
Erythrocyte sedimentation rate	Chemistry group, calcium and phosphate
	Serum or urine electrophoresis
	Urinalysis
	PSA

CBC – myeloma, infection
ESR – infection
Peripheral blood smear – lymphoma, leukemia, infection
Chemistry, calcium, phosphate – metabolic disease, diabetes, metastasis
Serum or urine electrophoresis – myeloma
Urinalysis – renal cell

Round cell lesions by age

Lesion	Age
Neuroblastoma	2 - 3
Eosinophilic granuloma	4 - 20
Ewing's sarcoma	10 - 25
Lymphoma	30 - 60
Myeloma	50 +
Metastasis	50 +
Infection	Any

Peri-articular tumors
Giant cell tumor
Chondroblastoma
Clear cell chondrosarcoma

5 Lesions that can look like anything
Fibrous dysplasia
Metastatic lesions
Chondroid lesions
Infection
Eosinophilic granuloma

Lodwick's Classification (radiographs of bone lesions)
IA. Well circumscribed, sclerotic
IB. Circumscribed, minimally sclerotic
IC. Poorly circumscribed
II. Moth eaten
III. Permeative

Malignant bone lesions
Myeloma
Lymphoma
Ewing's sarcoma
Metastatic lesions
Chondrosarcoma
Osteosarcoma
Chordoma
Adamantinoma

Malignant Soft tissue lesions
Soft tissue sarcoma
Fibrosarcoma
Liposarcoma
Leimyosarcoma
Malignant fibrous histiocytoma
Neurosarcoma
Rhabdomyosarcoma
Synovial sarcoma, Vascular sarcoma

Musculoskeletal Tumor Society (MSTS) Stages of Disease

Benign Disease	Malignant Disease
1 Benign, inactive	I Low grade
2 Benign, active	II High grade
3 Benign, aggressive	III With regional or distant metastasis

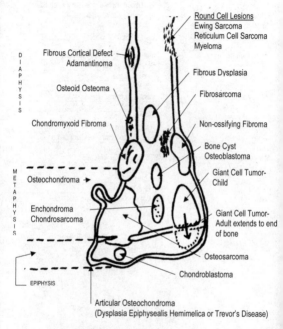

Redrawn with permission Madewell JE, Ragsdale BD, Sweet DE. Radiologic and pathologic analysis of solitary bone lesions, Part 1. Internal margins. Radiol Clin North Am 1981;19(4):785-814.

Steroid Preparations

Solubility	Generic Name	Trade Name	Equivalent Dose (mg)*
Most soluble	Betamethasone sodium phosphate	Celestone	0.6
Soluble	Dexamethasone sodium phosphate	Decadron	0.75
	Prednisolone sodium phosphate	Hydeltrasol	5
Slightly soluble	Prednisolone tebutate	Prednisol TBA	5
	Triamcinolone triacetate	Aristospan Forte	4
	Methylprednisone acetate	Depo-medrol	4
Relatively insoluble	Dexamethasone acetate	Decadron-LA	0.75
	Hydrocortisone acetate	Hydro-acetone	20
	Prednisolone acetate	Predalone	5
	Triamcinilone acetonide	Kenalog	4
Combination	Triamcinilone hexacetonide	Aristospan	4
	Betamethasone sodium phosphate-Betamethasone acetate[1]	Celestone soluspan	0.6

*For example, 0.6 mg of Betamethasone sodium phosphate is equivalent to 0.75 mg of Dexamethasone sodium phosphate, which is equivalent to 5 mg of prednisolone.
[1]Betamethasone acetate is slightly soluble
Used with permission Fadale PD, Wiggins ME. Corticosteroid Injections: Their Use and Abuse. JAAOS. 1994;2(3):133-139.

Journals

American Journal of Sports Medicine - www.sportsmed.org/journal/Default.htm
Arthroscopy – www.arthroscopyjournal.org
Clinical Orthopaedic and Related Research - www.corronline.com
Journal of Hand Surgery - www.worldscientific.com/journals/hs/hs.html
Journal of the American Academy of Orthopaedic Surgeons - www.jaaos.org
Orthopedics Today - www.orthopedicstoday.com
Seminars in Musculoskeletal Radiology – www.thieme.com
Spine - www.spinejournal.com
The Journal of Bone and Joint Surgery - www.jbjs.org
The Journal of Foot & Ankle Surgery - www.jfas.com
The Journal of Trauma - www.jtrauma.com
The Physician and Sportsmedicine   - www.physsportsmed.com

Companies

Biomet - www.biomet.com
DePuy/ACE - www.depuy.com
Howmedica - www.howmedica.com
Industry Link (various other companies) www.slackinc.com/bone/ortoday/otmall.asp
Instrument Maker, Inc - www.instmak.com
Johnson & Johnson – www.johnsonandjohnson.com
Lippincott – www.lww.com
Orthofix - www.orthofix.com
Smith & Nephew - www.sn-e.com
Tarascon Publishing – www.tarascon.com
WB Saunders - www.harcourt-international.com
Wright - www.WMT.com
Zimmer - www.zimmer.com

Orthopedic Web Sites

American Academy of Orthopedic Surgery - www.aaos.org
Orthopedic Medicine - www.orthopedics.about.com
SLACK Orthopedic Internet Directory -www.orthopedicstoday.com
Orthopaedic Database - www.ORTHOGUIDE.com

General Web Sites

U.S. Centers for Disease Control – www.cdc.gov
U.S. National Library of Medicine – www.nlm.nih.gov
National Inst. of Health – www.nih.gov
NIH Library – www.ncrr.nih.gov

Index

Page left blank for notes

Page left blank for notes

Page left blank for notes

Ordering Books From Tarascon Publishing

FAX	PHONE	INTERNET	MAIL
Fax credit card orders 24 hrs/day toll free to **877.929.9926**	For phone orders or customer service, call **800.929.9926**	Order through our OnLine store with your credit card at **www.tarascon.com**	Mail order & check to: **Tarascon Publishing PO Box 1159 Loma Linda, CA 92354**

Name

Address

City		State	Zip

Please send me:	Number	Price ‡
Tarascon Pocket Pharmacopoeia, Classic Shirt-Pocket Edition		$
Tarascon Pocket Pharmacopoeia, Deluxe Labcoat Pocket Edition		$
Tarascon Pocket Orthopaedica		$
Tarascon Internal Medicine & Critical Care Pocketbook		$
Tarascon Adult Emergency Pocketbook		$
Tarascon Pediatric Emergency Pocketbook		$
How to be a Truly Excellent Junior Medical Student		$

‡ Price per Copy by Number of Copies Ordered						
Total # of each ordered	1–9	10–49	50-99	≥100	**Subtotal**	$
Pocket Pharmacop Classic	$8.95	$7.95	$6.95	$5.95		
Pocket Pharmacop Deluxe	$17.95	$15.25	$13.45	$12.55	**California**	$
Pocket Orthopaedica	$11.95	$9.90	$8.95	$8.35	**only add**	
Internal Med Pocketbook	$11.95	$9.90	$8.95	$8.35	**7.5%**	
Adult Emerg Pocketbook	$11.95	$9.90	$8.95	$8.35	**sales tax**	
Peds Emerg Pocketbook	$9.95	$8.25	$7.45	$6.95	**Shipping**	$
How...Truly Excellent JMS	$9.95	$8.25	$7.45	$6.95	**and**	

Shipping & Handling					handling (table)	
If subtotal is →	<$10	$10-24	$25-99	$100-300		
Standard shipping	$1.00	$2.50	$5.00	$8.00		$
UPS 2-day air*	$12.00	$12.00	$14.00	$18.00	**TOTAL**	

*No post office boxes

☐ **Charge credit card**:	☐ VISA ☐ Mastercard ☐ American Express
Card number	Exp Date
Signature	E-mail	Phone